Osteoporosis Management

Editor: I.R. Reid

Adis International

Auckland • Buenos Aires • Chester • Hong Kong • Madrid • Milan • Osaka • Paris • Philadelphia • São Paulo • Sydney

Osteoporosis Management

Editor: I.R. Reid

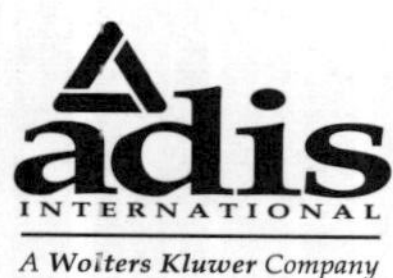

Commercial Manager: Gordon Mallarkey
Publication Manager: Lorna Venter-Lewis
Adis International Limited
 ISBN 0-86471-083-6

Earlier versions of some articles in this book were published in Adis International's peer-reviewed medical journals. The editor has collated the articles and worked with the authors to adapt and update the information for this publication.

Printed in Hong Kong.

Foreword

In the last 20 years, osteoporosis has moved from being regarded as an inevitable part of growing old to being recognised as a specific medical condition, amenable to diagnosis and treatment. Several different forces have brought about this transformation. The progressive ageing of our community has hugely increased the number of osteoporotic fractures that are occurring, providing the incentive to address the problem. Furthermore, the advent of bone densitometry has permitted the systematic study of the development of osteoporosis, and demonstrated that fracture risk can be quantified. Finally, bone densitometry has made possible the carrying out of clinical studies necessary for the evaluation of existing pharmaceutical agents and for the development of new ones. Much of this development has occurred in the last 10 years, and has resulted in our having a substantial and rapidly expanding knowledge base regarding the efficacy of osteoporotic medications.

It is timely, therefore, to review this knowledge and to consider areas of likely expansion and development in the future. This book addresses this need, and I hope will provide a broad introduction to the topic for those who are new to the field, while at the same time being thought provoking for those already familiar with the problems and challenges of the osteoporotic patient.

Ian R Reid, MD
Auckland, New Zealand

Osteoporosis Management

Contents

Pharmacological Management of Osteoporosis in Postmenopausal Women

A Comparative Review

Ian R. Reid

Department of Medicine, University of Auckland, Auckland, New Zealand

Osteoporosis is a condition characterised by reduced bone mass and usually associated with the micro-architectural deterioration of bone. The latter term refers to the development of perforations within trabecular plates and, ultimately, to the complete loss of trabecular elements. Some individuals are more at risk of developing osteoporosis because the peak skeletal mass they attained following puberty was low, but an almost invariable contributor to the development of both low bone mass and micro-architectural deterioration, is the substantial increase in bone resorption that occurs after the menopause. This results from a reduction in circulating estrogen levels. The precise mechanism by which estrogens reduces bone resorption remains a matter of controversy. It may act directly on the osteoclast to promote apoptosis[1] but its major effect is probably through regulation of the production of osteolytic cytokines such as interleukin(IL)-1, IL-6 and tumour necrosis factor-α from stromal and mononuclear cells in the bone marrow.[2] Estrogens may also increase bone marrow levels of osteoprotegerin, a peptide which inhibits osteoclast development.[3]

The definition of osteoporosis is arbitrary since bone density and fracture risk are both continuous variables, an individual's value for which will change substantially throughout their lifespan. In the past, this fact has been partially obscured by defining osteoporosis either as the occurrence of a fracture after minimal trauma or, the more recent World Health Organization definition, as a bone density which is more than 2.5 standard deviations below the mean normal value for young women (i.e. T-score <-2.5).[4] Such definitions may meet the needs of epidemiological and regulatory agencies more used to dealing with infectious or neoplastic diseases. However, they are of only limited value to clinicians making decisions regarding therapy. Such decisions will be based on a global assessment of an individual's future risk of fractures, balanced with the efficacy, tolerability, safety and cost of the available interventions. Since cost, in particular, can change substantially over time (e.g. as a result of patent expiration), thresholds for intervention can also change substantially as a result of such completely non-biological factors. Furthermore, definitions based entirely on bone density measurements produce disparate results depending on the skeletal site and technique of bone density measurement, and their application to individuals other than Caucasian females has yet to be addressed.

The prevention of osteoporosis is essentially the prevention of fractures. The frequency of fractures will reflect the balance of skeletal strength and the intensity of skeletal trauma. Thus, measures aimed towards the optimisation of the former and the minimisation of the latter are potentially important in the management of osteoporosis. Reductions in skeletal trauma can be achieved by falls prevention and by the minimisation of skeletal loading following falls. Several falls prevention programmes have been demonstrated to be effective in the elderly,[5,6] and the maintenance of moderate exercise levels is probably important to this end. There is preliminary evidence that the use of hip protectors can reduce fracture rates [7] and the use of shock-absorbing surfaces in the home, particularly on floors, may also be important.

While skeletal strength can be manipulated pharmacologically, it is also subject to other influences. Bodyweight, particularly fat mass, has a major impact on bone mineral density (BMD), so the maintenance of bodyweight is pivotal. Smoking results in 5 to 10% reductions in BMD. Very high alcohol intakes (particularly in men) may also be deleterious, though the evidence is inconsistent in women. The maintenance of normal estrogen production throughout the reproductive years is important for the optimisation of bone mass, and postmenopausal women with a history of delayed menarche, oligo/amenorrhoea or premature menopause have reduced BMD. Exercise has a modest effect on BMD but the role of diet remains unclear, since the putative dietary risk factors (low intakes of calcium and colecalciferol, and high intakes of caffeine, sodium and protein) have not been consistently demonstrated to influence BMD in cross-sectional population studies. Despite uncertainty relating to some of these factors, there is a general consensus that patients at risk of osteoporosis should be encouraged to stop smoking, to maintain moderate levels of exercise that do not involve severe skeletal loading, to maintain bodyweight (eg, above 60 kgs if possible), to have a calcium intake greater than 1000 to 1500 mg/day, to maintain normal serum levels of calcifidiol (25-hydroxyvitamin D), and to moderate alcohol and caffeine intakes (e.g. to no more than 4 drinks of each per day). Such modifications will produce only modest changes in BMD so that pharmacological interventions are necessary in individuals with a high fracture risk.[8] The available pharmacological interventions will now be reviewed.

1. Calcium

Calcium is the principal mineral constituent of bone and its supply during skeletal growth may be a limiting factor in the attainment of peak bone mass. Throughout life, there are obligatory losses of calcium in both urine and faeces. Since the levels of this mineral in the extracellular fluid are tightly regulated, when calcium losses are not met by dietary calcium intake, secretion of parathyroid hormone increases and the calcium necessary to maintain normal circulating levels is mobilised from the skeleton. For these reasons, it has been postulated that the provision of additional calcium may reduce bone loss in postmenopausal women.

This question has been addressed through a large number of observational studies which have produced conflicting results.[9] However, the data from randomised controlled trials are much more consistent, demonstrating a benefit to BMD of 0.5 to 1% over periods of 2 to 4 years as a result of the use of calcium supplementation.[10-16] The beneficial effect is seen throughout the skeleton. It may be more marked in late postmenopausal women,[13] in individuals with a lower baseline calcium intake,[13] and with the use of more bioavailable calcium preparations.[13,17] In skeletal sites rich in trabecular bone, much of the benefit associated with calcium supplementation appears to occur within the first few months of treatment, suggesting that the effect represents a remodelling transient rather than a sustained change in bone balance. However, we have demonstrated a sustained reduction in the rate of total body bone loss in healthy postmenopausal women, suggesting a long term alteration in the balance of cortical bone (fig. 1). This pattern of change suggests that calcium supplementation might result in reduced rates of fracture, and such a reduction in fracture rate has now been demonstrated in three relatively small studies of calcium supplementation.[10,16,18] However, there remains a need for a much larger definitive study before the anti-fracture efficacy of calcium supplements can really be accepted.

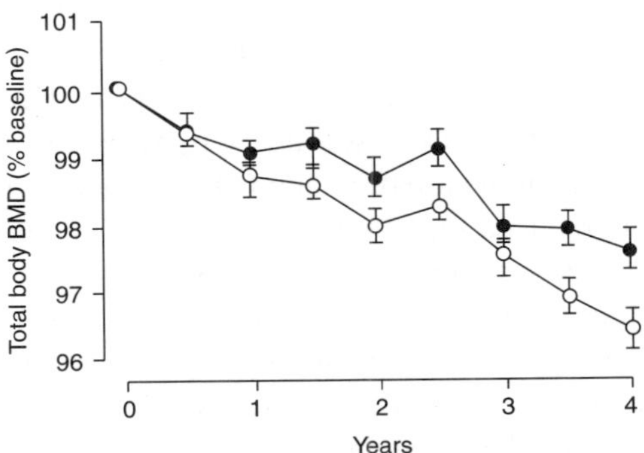

Fig. 1. Total body bone mineral density (BMD) in postmenopausal women treated with calcium (1 g/day) or placebo for 4 years. The results are given as mean ± sem and are expressed as a percentage of baseline values. Loss of BMD was significantly greater in the placebo group (reproduced from Reid et al.,[16] with permission).

Calcium may have an important role as an adjunct to other therapies. Nieves et al.[19] have recently reviewed studies of estrogen treatment of postmenopausal women and found that in those studies in which calcium was given together with estrogens the increase in bone density was greater than with estrogens alone. This is consistent with the prospective controlled study of Ettinger et al.[20] and the recent observational study of Davis et al.[21]

Calcium is generally well tolerated, although it causes constipation in some individuals. Its use may be associated with a small increase in the risk of kidney stones[22] but it has been suggested to reduce the risk of colorectal cancer, and to reduce blood pressure and serum lipid levels.

Most authorities recommend that postmenopausal women maintain a calcium intake of 1000 to 1500 mg/day, equivalent to 4 to 6 servings of dairy products. In those who would prefer to take their calcium in the form of a supplement, daily doses of 500 to 1000mg are usually given to achieve a total calcium intake within or slightly above this target range. It should be noted that a calcium supplement of 500 to 1000 mg/day (often with a vitamin D preparation) is given to all participants in many clinical trials, and so forms the comparator therapy in most of the studies described subsequently in this review.

2. Vitamin D (Cholecalciferol)

Vitamin D (cholecalciferol) is produced in the skin as a result of the action of ultraviolet light on 7-dehydrocholesterol. Vitamin D itself is virtually inactive biologically, but much of the parent compound is converted to calcifidiol (25-hydroxyvitamin D) in the liver. This is the principal form in the circulation, where it is bound to vitamin D-binding globulin. The final stage in the bioactivation of vitamin D occurs in the kidney where calcifidiol is further hydroxylated to form calcitriol (1,25-dihydroxyvitamin D). This is 1000 times more active than its immediate precursor and its production is under tight homeostatic control. It circulates in concentrations approximately 0.1% of those of calcifidiol, and is bound to the same carrier protein.

In vitamin D deficiency, serum levels of calcifidiol fall, resulting indirectly in elevations of parathyroid hormone which maintains serum calcium by mobilising calcium from bone and also by increasing 1α-hydroxylation of calcifidiol to calcitriol. Thus, mild to moderate vitamin D deficiency leads to secondary hyperparathyroidism and accelerated bone loss. This is the rationale for the use of vitamin D supplementation in the elderly or in any other individuals in whom reduced sunlight exposure has led to reduced concentrations of this pro-hormone.

When considering the use of vitamin D supplements to produce 'normal' levels of this compound, it is important to consider not only what is normal but what is optimal. This has recently been addressed by Malabanan et al.[23] in a study of the effect of vitamin D supplementation on circulating levels of parathyroid hormone. It was demonstrated that vitamin D supplementation suppressed parathyroid hormone levels only in individuals whose baseline serum calcifidiol levels were <50 nmol/L. If this preliminary observation is confirmed in larger studies, it would suggest that 50 nmol/L is a more appropriate target level for calcifidiol when supplementing with vitamin D, than the lower end of the 'normal range', which is influenced by the fact that many individuals in the elderly population have suboptimal vitamin D status.

Physiological supplements of calciferol (e.g. 400 IU/day) reduce parathyroid hormone levels and lead to increases in bone density, particularly at the femoral neck.[24,25] Two large studies have assessed the effect on fracture rates of calciferol supplementation alone. Lips et al.[26] showed no change in fracture incidence in 2578 men and women over the age of 70 years randomised to calciferol 400 IU/day or placebo, whereas Heikinheimo et al.[27] showed that 150 000IU of vitamin D annually reduced symptomatic fracture rates by 25% in a cohort of 800 elderly individuals in Finland. At least two further major studies have been reported in which calcium was coadministered with calciferol to elderly individuals. Chapuy et al.[28,29] demonstrated a reduction of more than one quarter in nonvertebral and hip fracture rates in a cohort of 3000 elderly women studied over a period of 3 years. Dawson-Hughes et al.[30] demonstrated a reduction of nonvertebral fracture rates by more than one half in 400 older men and women randomised to calcium 500 mg/day plus 700 IU/day vitamin D, or to placebo. It is not possible to determine whether the calcium, the vitamin D or the combination were the essential components to the success of these two studies, but they do point to the possibility of a major reduction in morbidity in elderly patients as a result of a well tolerated and inexpensive intervention.

Vitamin D supplementation seems to produce no benefit in early postmenopausal women who are already vitamin D replete.[31,32] Its use as a physiological supplement is fundamentally different from the use of high dose calciferol or 1α-hydroxylated vitamin D metabolites to pharmacologically manipulate intestinal calcium absorption. Both of these strategies bypass the normal homeostatic controls of vitamin D metabolism and therefore carry a significant risk of hypercalcaemia and hypercalciuria. The use of pharmacological doses of calciferol has not been demonstrated to confer any beneficial effects on bone density.[33] The effects of 1α-hydroxylated compounds on bone density will be discussed in section 7.

In conclusion, suboptimal vitamin D status is very common in the elderly, mainly because of reduced sunlight exposure. Its prevention is straightforward, well tolerated and inexpensive, and appears to produce substantial benefits to fracture rates.

3. Hormone Replacement Therapy

The pivotal role of reduced circulating levels of estrogen in the genesis of postmenopausal bone loss suggested that estrogen replacement was likely to be a successful therapy. This was first explored in detail by Lindsay et al.[34,35] In that study of women undergoing oophorectomy, participants were randomised to treatment with estrogens or placebo and follow-up continued for 15 years (fig. 2). Bone loss at the metacarpal was completely prevented by estrogen replacement, whereas nearly one-third of baseline bone mineral was lost in the placebo group. Over the first 9 years of the study, women receiving placebo gained 3.2kg in bodyweight, lost 0.9cm in height and had an average of 1.6 vertebral deformities, whereas there was no significant change in any of these indices in the individuals receiving estrogens.[34] These beneficial effects of estrogens on bone have now been confirmed in healthy women 5 to 10 years after the menopause,[36,37] in those in their seventies[38] as well as in those with established osteoporosis.[39-41] The study of Lufkin et al.[39] indicated that the number of new fractures was decreased by half after only 12 months of therapy, and a large number of observational studies suggest that long term use of estrogens is also associated with a reduced incidence of nonvertebral fractures, particularly hip fractures.[42,43] These studies suggest that current use of hormone replacement therapy (HRT) reduces fracture risk by as much as 70% and past use by about half that amount. Bone density is significantly increased, and vertebral fracture risk and height loss substantially reduced in long term users of HRT.[44,45]

Following the cessation of HRT, bone loss recommences, probably at about the same rate as in individuals who have not taken HRT.[46] Therefore, there is a waning of the protective effect from this medication, such that use in the years immediately after the menopause may leave very little residual benefit 20 to 30 years later when an individual's fracture risk is highest.[47] While long term use of estrogens from the menopause into old age appears to maximise bone density,[44,48] the initiation of therapy after the age of 60 years appears to produce nearly comparable benefits to bone density[48] and may be associated with a lower risk of breast cancer.

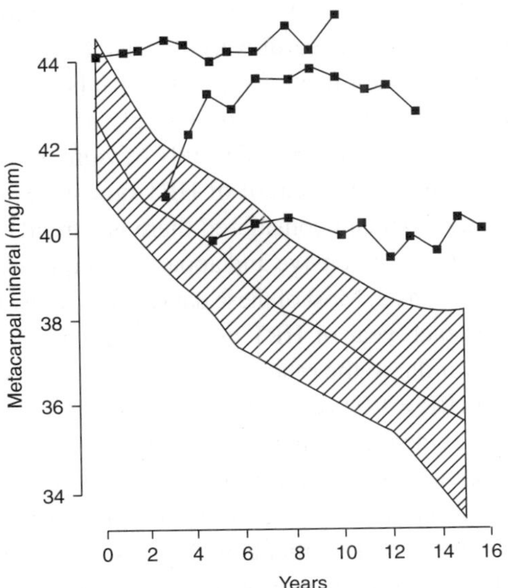

Fig. 2. The effects of estrogen replacement therapy (ERT) on metacarpal bone mineral content in women who had undergone ovariectomy. In the groups receiving ERT, the intervals between ovariectomy and the introduction of ERT are indicated on the x-axis. The loss of bone in those receiving placebo is indicated by the hatched region (reproduced from Lindsay,[35] with permission).

The formulation of estrogens used, and the route and schedule of administration do not appear to influence their effect on bone. Thus, conjugated estrogens 0.625mg orally are equivalent to estradiol 1 to 2 mg/day orally, or to 17β estradiol 50 μg/day transdermally. Opinion is divided as to whether progestogens have an additive effect to that of estrogens,[37,49] although norethisterone probably does, partly because of its estrogenic and androgenic actions.[50] Tibolone is closely related to norethisterone and has effects on bone density comparable with those of estrogens or combined HRT.[51] In hysterectomised women, estrogens can be given alone, but in those with an intact uterus they are usually combined with a progestogen to prevent endometrial hyperplasia and an increased risk of endometrial cancer. Progestogens can be given cyclically (e.g. medroxyprogesterone 5 mg/day for 12 to 14 days/ month) but, after the perimenopause, estrogens and progestogens are more commonly given continuously (e.g. 1 of the above estrogen doses plus medroxyprogesterone 2.5 mg/day or norethisterone 1 mg/day) since this results in amenorrhoea in more than 80% of patients receiving long term therapy.

The role of HRT use in combination with other agents is now beginning to be explored. There is evidence that its combination with bisphosphonates,[52-54] calcitriol[55] and fluoride [56] all result in greater increases in bone density than are produced by the individual agents alone.

3.1 Other Effects of Estrogens

There is clear evidence from randomised controlled trials in postmenopausal women that HRT improves indices of cardiovascular risk, particularly lipid profiles. Prospective controlled studies in animals have also demonstrated that HRT substantially reduces the development of atheroma, and there are extensive observational data from humans supporting this contention. The latter data must be interpreted with caution as users of HRT frequently have a reduced prevalence of other cardiovascular risk factors.[57] At the present time there are no adequately powered, randomised, controlled trials assessing cardiovascular end-points in healthy postmenopausal women. Surprisingly, the recently published Heart and Estrogen/Progestin Replacement Study (HERS) study of women with pre-existing ischaemic heart disease, failed to demonstrate any benefit of HRT on cardiovascular event rates, although if years 2 to 4 of the study alone are considered there is a trend to fewer events in those receiving HRT.[58]

There is an extensive and apparently contradictory literature concerning the effects of HRT on breast cancer. Most of these data have recently been meta-analysed.[59] This analysis suggests that for each year of HRT use the relative risk (RR) of having breast cancer is increased by 1.023, similar to the relative risk for each year of increased age at the menopause in never-users of HRT (RR = 1.028). Cancers diagnosed in users of HRT tended to be less advanced and there was no evidence of an effect on mortality. In Western countries, the cumulative incidence of breast cancer between the ages of 50 and 70 years in never-users of HRT is approximately 45 per thousand. In this context, the use of HRT for 5, 10 or 15 years would be expected to produce a further 2, 6 or 12 patients with breast cancer, respectively.

HRT also produces effects on a number of other end-points. It decreases hot flushes, is protective against urogenital atrophy, may be protective against dermal atrophy, leads to an approximately 3-fold increase in risk of thromboembolic events but may reduce the risk of colon cancer. Thus, it is an effective therapy for the prevention and treatment of postmenopausal osteoporosis but decisions about its use require a complex balancing of a large number of issues.

4. Selective Estrogen Receptor Modulators

The selective estrogen receptor modulators (SERMs) are a new class of agents which have come into existence following the discovery that tamoxifen, an estrogen receptor antagonist, paradoxically produced estrogen-like effects on both bone and lipid metabolism.[60-62] The possibility that this class of compounds could also be used for the prevention of breast cancer has led to an explosion of interest. However, tamoxifen acts as an estrogen agonist in the endometrium, probably increasing the risk of endometrial cancer. This has led to the development of other SERMs which lack agonist effects at this site.

At present, raloxifene is the only other SERM which has been studied in long term clinical trials and which is available for therapeutic use. Raloxifene in the commonly used dosages of 60 mg/day and 120 mg/day, has effects similar to low dosages of estrogens in that it reduces indices of bone turnover by 10 to 30% and increases spinal bone density by 1 to 3% over 1 to 2 years.[63,64] Results from the Multiple Outcomes of Raloxifene Evaluation (MORE) study, involving 7705 women with osteoporosis, indicate that raloxifene use is associated with a halving of the risk of vertebral fractures but no significant decrease in that of nonvertebral fractures (RR 0.91).[65] This study has also demonstrated a 76% reduction in the incidence of breast cancer but an increased risk of thromboembolic disease comparable with that seen with HRT.[66] No significant effect on cardiovascular end-points has yet been demonstrated, although there is a downward trend in the interim data.

The precise mechanism of action of the SERMs remains to be elucidated. They appear to bind to the estrogen receptor but, on binding, to produce different conformational changes in the receptor from those produced by estradiol itself. A number of other accessary proteins appear to be involved in the binding of the estrogen receptor to DNA, and the distribution of these accessary proteins varies from tissue to tissue. This may account for the tissue-specific agonist-antagonist effects observed with these agents.

The role of SERMs in the postmenopause remains to be determined. They may have a useful role in the prevention of osteoporosis but the fact that their effects on bone mass are smaller than those of either HRT or the bisphosphonates, and that their efficacy in preventing nonvertebral fractures has not been established, makes them less attractive in patients at high fracture risk. If their efficacy in preventing breast cancer is confirmed, then they may become much more widely used for this indication. A number of new SERMs are under development and these agents will help to define the place of this group in this area of therapeutics.

5. Bisphosphonates

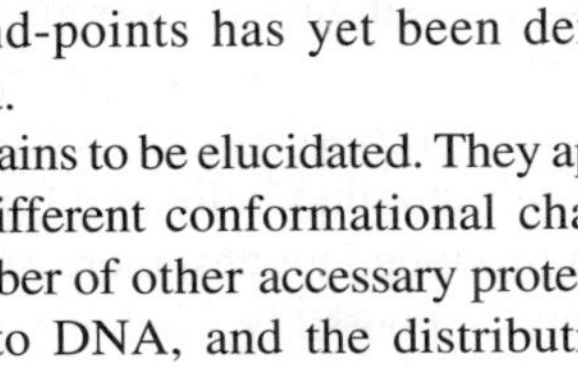

The bisphosphonate nucleus is illustrated in figure 3. It consists of two phosphate groups linked through a central carbon atom. This structure is extremely stable in biological systems, and binds avidly to exposed mineral surfaces as a result of the negative charges on the phosphate groups. By substitution at the two variable groups on the central

Fig. 3. The bisphosphonate nucleus. Substitution of R′ and R″ creates the different members of the family, which differ in their antiresorptive potency and adverse effects. All have the two phosphate groups giving high affinity for bone mineral, and the P-C-P bond which confers its high stability.

carbon atom, a wide variety of different bisphosphonates can be manufactured. The principal action of the bisphosphonates on bone metabolism is to inhibit osteoclastic resorption. Current indications are that at least two different mechanisms are involved.[67,68] Clodronate and etidronate substitute for pyrophosphate in the formation of ATP, disrupting energy metabolism within cells. Most of the other bisphosphonates appear to block the production of compounds in the mevalonate pathway which are important for the binding of some proteins to the plasma membrane (prenylation of proteins). This leads to the disruption of a variety of cellular processes. The marked *in vivo* specificity of the bisphosphonates to osteoclasts probably arises from their physicochemical targeting to bone and their subsequent ingestion by osteoclasts at the time of bone resorption.

Since the publication of the first randomised controlled trial of bisphosphonates in osteoporosis management in 1988,[69] there has been an avalanche of further information documenting their safety and efficacy in a variety of bone diseases, including postmenopausal osteoporosis. The studies of Storm et al.[70] and Watts et al.[71] using cyclical etidronate (400 mg/day for 2 weeks, repeated every 3 months) indicated that this regimen produced modest increases in bone density and possibly a halving of the number of vertebral fractures. More recently, a number of large studies with the more potent aminobisphosphonate, alendronate, have been published.[72,73] These demonstrate reductions in biochemical indices of bone resorption to the levels seen in premenopausal women, increases in lumbar spine bone density of about 8% at 3 years,[72] and a reduction in the risk of hip, vertebral and forearm fractures of almost 50% (fig. 4).[73] Similar bone density changes have been demonstrated with a variety of other bisphosphonates and administration regimens. Quantitative histomorphometry of bone in patients treated with alendronate shows diminished depth of erosion cavities and a diminished activation frequency, but no evidence of abnormal mineralisation.[74]

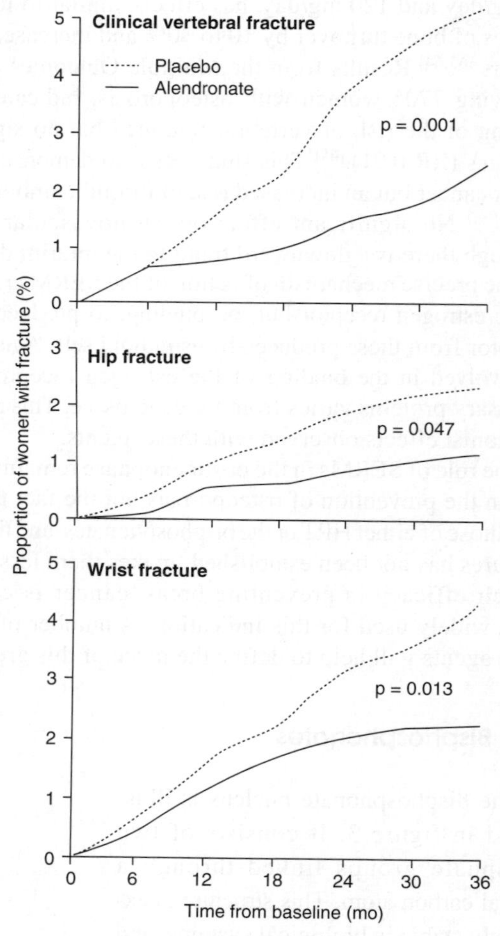

Fig. 4. Cumulative proportions of women with fractures according to treatment with placebo or alendronate (5 mg/day for 2 years, followed by 10 mg/day in year 3). Patients had a low femoral neck bone density and an existing vertebral fracture at trial entry (reproduced from Black et al.,[73] with permission).

The bisphosphonates are generally well tolerated, although the aminobisphosphonates sometimes cause upper gastrointestinal irritation. There are reports of this problem with both pamidronate[75] and alendronate,[76-78] although in the randomised controlled osteoporosis treatment trials of the latter agent there was no evidence of significant gastrointestinal adverse effects. This may be because patients with significant upper gastrointestinal disease did not enter the studies, or because administration regimens were more strictly adhered to in the disciplined environment of a clinical trial. Reports of oesophageal ulceration have been a particular concern, and probably result from reflux of bisphosphonate tablets into the oesophagus from the stomach. To circumvent this potential problem, aminobisphosphonates should be taken with a full glass of water and the patient should remain upright over the next hour. All agents in this class have very low solubility and will bind to any positively charged ion. Therefore, they should be taken fasting with water alone, and at least half an hour before any other food or fluid. Antacids and mineral supplements, in particular, should be avoided at the time of bisphosphonate administration.

The bisphosphonates have provided a major alternative in both the treatment and the prevention of postmenopausal and other osteoporoses. Their effectiveness appears to be comparable to that of HRT and, since they only have significant actions on bone, decisions regarding their use are much more straightforward than are those regarding HRT. Their long residence time in bone makes the use of intermittent regimens viable, and new agents which can be given by bolus injection at intervals of 3 or more months are likely to become a reality in the next few years.

6. Thiazide Diuretics

The use of thiazide diuretics is associated with reduced urinary calcium excretion, and some observational studies indicate that users of thiazide diuretics have increased bone mass and a reduced risk of hip fracture.[79] However, these findings might be accounted for by higher bodyweight and higher bone mass in patients with hypertension, the principal group using thiazide diuretics. Two preliminary reports have recently been published of randomised controlled trials of thiazide diuretics in healthy older women, which have documented beneficial effects on bone density of about 1% over treatment periods of 2 to 3 years.[80,81] These small effects may result in effects on bone density which are large enough to influence fracture risk with long term use. Thus, like calcium, thiazide diuretics may have a role as a widely used preventative intervention, but they are clearly not adequate as a monotherapy for established osteoporosis.

7. Vitamin D Metabolites

With the discovery that the 1α-hydroxylation of vitamin D greatly increased its potency, came an interest in using this compound pharmacologically to increase intestinal calcium absorption as a means of treating osteoporosis. Such an approach would only be effective if intestinal calcium absorption was a critical contributor to the development of osteoporosis, something which has never been established. When using these compounds (calcitriol or alfacalcidol) in treating osteoporosis, their other principal activity, that of stimulating osteoclastic bone resorption, needs to also be borne in mind, since this could result in reduced bone mass. Thus, the theoretical case for the use of these agents in osteoporosis is dubious since it could be argued that they could cause either benefit or harm, and they clearly carry the risk of inducing hypercalciuria and hypercalcaemia.

Clinical studies have not yet resolved the question of their value in osteoporosis therapy. Studies in Danish women in their 50s[82] and their 70s[38,83] showed no beneficial effects of calcitriol on bone loss, and suggested that it accelerated the rate of vertebral height loss. Similar negative findings have been reported in women with osteoporosis by Falch et al.[84] and by Ott and Chestnut.[85] In contrast, Gallagher and Goldgar[86] and Aloia et al.[87] observed small increases in total body BMD in patients with osteoporosis treated with calcitriol.

A strong boost to the case for using calcitriol for treating osteoporosis came from the study of Tilyard et al.[88] which documented the occurrence of fewer fractures in patients receiving this therapy compared with those treated with calcium alone. However, the number of patients with new fractures was stable over the 3 years of the study in patients receiving calcitriol, whereas it showed a 3-fold increase in those receiving calcium. This pattern of response to calcium supplementation has not been observed in other studies and suggests there is something atypical about this group of patients treated with calcium which renders them unsuitable as a reliable comparator.

There is a similar inconsistency in the data with alfacalcidol (reviewed in Reid[89]) though the observation that a number of positive studies have come from Italy and Japan has led to a suggestion that there may be racial differences in responsiveness to these agents. Such differences could be related to differences in customary dietary calcium intakes or to differences in vitamin D receptor gene alleles. However, 2 recent negative studies from each of these countries[90,91] cast doubt upon the need to invoke such explanations.

Several recent studies have suggested that vitamin D metabolites may have a role as an adjunctive therapy when given with an antiresorptive agent. Such a combination has a theoretical appeal since coadministration of these agents with HRT or a bisphosphonate will minimise their capacity for stimulating bone resorption while leaving their beneficial effects on intestinal calcium absorption intact. Frediani et al.,[92] Masud et al.[93] and Gutteridge et al.[55] have demonstrated beneficial effects from the addition of calcitriol to alendronate, etidronate and HRT, respectively.

Thus, the role of the 1α-hydroxylated metabolites of vitamin D in the management of osteoporosis remains uncertain. Since the data relating to HRT and the bisphosphonates are much more consistently positive, use for these latter agents as first line therapies has a much sounder basis.

8. Calcitonin

Calcitonin is a peptide hormone secreted from the C cells of the thyroid, which directly inhibits osteoclastic bone resorption. Until recently, it was administered by injection, but there are now intranasal preparations available. Its effects on BMD have been assessed in a large number of relatively small studies many of which have shown beneficial effects,[94] although not all.[90,95]

Recently, preliminary findings of the Prevent Recurrence of Osteoporotic Fractures (PROOF) study have been published. This is by far the largest study of calcitonin use. 1255 women with established osteoporosis were randomised to placebo or to intranasal salmon calcitonin in dosages of 100, 200 or 400 U/day. At 3 years there were no significant differences between the groups in BMD[96] and at 5 years there was a significant reduction in risk of vertebral fracture in patients receiving the 200 U/day dosage (RR 0.64) but no significant effect with the other 2 dosages.[97] The number of hip fractures was halved in the patients receiving any dosage of calcitonin, but this effect was not significant. The long term use of calcitonin is associated with the development of neutralising antibodies in some patients and with the down-regulation of calcitonin receptors, which might account for the relatively disappointing results of this long term study.

As with the vitamin D metabolites, the inconsistency of these studies and the absence of the clear establishment of antifracture efficacy militate against calcitonin being regarded as a first line therapy for osteoporosis.

9. Fluoride

It has been known since the 1960s that high fluoride concentrations in drinking water resulted in marked increases in bone density (skeletal fluorosis). The administration of fluoride to patients with osteoporosis has been demonstrated to produce substantial increases in bone density, with annual rates of increase of spinal bone density as high as 8% sustained over up to 4 years.[98] Fluoride produces these effects by a direct anabolic effect on the osteoblast, possibly by increasing growth factor-induced tyrosine phosphorylation.[99]

However, sustained exposure to high levels of fluoride has a second effect on bone; it results in the incorporation of fluoride into the hydroxyapatite crystal with a resultant inhibition of bone mineralisation. This results in the development of osteomalacia, which may account for the fact that the studies in which the most marked increases in bone density have been demonstrated have not been associated with decreases in fracture rate.[98,100]

Some other studies have suggested that fluoride use is associated with a reduced fracture rate[101,102] and it is possible that these positive results are related to the use of different preparations or doses, although in the Fluoride and Vertebral Osteoporosis Study (FAVOS) neither of these variables was shown to influence outcome.[100] Until these positive studies can be consistently reproduced, fluoride is probably not appropriate for widespread use in osteoporosis treatment. The beneficial effects of fluoride on bone mass occur almost exclusively in trabecular bone so it is really only suitable for the management of vertebral osteoporosis – it may even accelerate bone loss at cortical sites. Because fluoride accumulates in the skeleton with continued used, periods of continuous therapy are usually limited to 3 to 4 years.

10. Anabolic Steroids

A class of therapeutic agents sometimes regarded as promoting new bone formation is the anabolic steroids. Those used in osteoporosis therapy are testosterone analogues modified to reduce their virilising effects. However, these modifications are only partially successful and the long term clinical use of these agents continues to be severely limited by the development of acne, hirsutism and voice changes, although they do produce changes in bone density comparable to those associated with HRT.[103] The extent to which they function as promoters of bone growth *in vivo* is uncertain, and some studies suggest their major action to be antiresorptive.

11. Selecting a Therapy

Although many therapies have been shown to have beneficial effects on bone density, not all these effects are equivalent. In general, HRT and the bisphosphonates cause the greatest increases in BMD, as is demonstrated in figure 5. This shows the effects of a variety of therapies studied in our unit and is typical of results found by many others. The data for the SERM

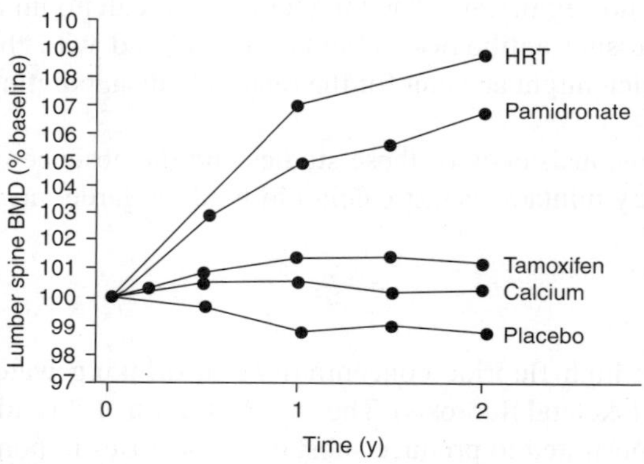

Fig. 5. Comparison of the effects of calcium (1 g/day), tamoxifen (20 mg/day), hormone replacement therapy (HRT) and the bisphosphonate pamidronate (150 mg/day), on lumbar spine bone mineral density (BMD) of postmenopausal women over 2 years' of therapy. The HRT and pamidronate groups also received calcium 1 g/day. The calcium and placebo groups were healthy women whereas the other individuals had at least 1 pre-existing vertebral fracture. The mean ages and BMD at baseline in the respective groups were: placebo: 58 years, 1.05 g/cm^2; calcium: 58 years, 1.02 g/cm^2; tamoxifen: 58 years, 1.09 g/cm^2; pamidronate: 65 years, 0.99 g/cm^2; HRT: 64 years, 0.83 g/cm^2. The figure is a compilation of separate studies carried out using the same densitometer over approximately the same time.[15,41,62,104]

tamoxifen are very similar to those for raloxifene, which also clearly has smaller effects on bone than HRT. Comparison of the antifracture efficacies of agents is difficult since the confidence intervals on the relative risk of fracture in the various studies are wide and much larger studies will be necessary before any differences between agents in this regard can be proven. In the meantime, it seems reasonable to rank the antiresorptive agents (i.e. bisphosphonates, HRT and SERMS) according to their effects on BMD.

As well as relative efficacy, the other effects of these agents are important considerations in an individual's choice of a therapy. Some of the important issues are highlighted in table I, and table II sets out the choices often made in commonly occurring situations. Often decisions will be based on subjective criteria, such as whether a patient is more concerned about her risk of breast cancer than that of heart disease.

12. Future Therapies

The development of new pharmaceuticals for the treatment of osteoporosis is the focus of much research effort at present. Unfortunately, a number of agents that have progressed the most have been found to have problems, either with adverse effects or insufficient efficacy.

Table I. Pros and cons of agents used in the management of postmenopausal osteoporosis

Agent	Pros	Cons
Calcium	Cheap, safe, accessible	Partial efficacy only
Hormone replacement therapy (HRT)	Antifracture efficacy, ?↓ CVD, relieves menopausal symptoms	?↑ Breast cancer risk
Raloxifene	Vertebral antifracture efficacy, ↓ breast cancer risk, well tolerated	Less effect on BMD than HRT, short term data only. ? effect on nonvertebral fracture
Bisphosphonates	Antifracture efficacy at hip spine and forearm. BMD effects comparable to HRT. Available parenterally	Data relatively short term, gastrointestinal adverse effects with alendronate
Calcitonin	Intranasal preparation now available	Efficacy uncertain
Thiazide diuretic	Cheap, safe. Antihypertensive	Partial efficacy only
Fluoride	↑↑ BMD	Mixed data regarding antifracture efficacy. Major effect at spine only
Calcitriol, alfacalcidol	Well tolerated	Efficacy uncertain, risk of hypercalcaemia and hypercalciuria
Anabolic steroids	↑ BMD and ? ↑ well-being	Virilising adverse effects

BMD = bone mineral density; **CVD** = cardiovascular disease; ↓ = decrease; ↑ = increase.

Table II. Choice of interventions in patients at risk of fractures

Age (y)	Fractures	T-Score	First-line intervention	Alternatives
50s	None	–1	Calcium, thiazide diuretic	HRT if has menopausal symptoms, raloxifene if at high risk of breast cancer
50s	None	–2	Calcium + HRT	BP, raloxifene
60s+	None	–3	Calcium + HRT or BP	Raloxifene or calcitonin if intolerant of both HRT and BPs
60s+	Yes	Any	As above	As above
60s+	Multiple	<–4	In patients with severe osteoporosis or in whom response to therapy is poor, consider multiple therapies e.g. HRT + BP, either or both + calcitriol	
80s+	Yes or No	Any	Assess vitamin D status and supplement with calciferol if necessary, in addition to any of above measures that are indicated	

BP = bisphosphonates; **HRT** = hormone replacement therapy.

Thus, it is unclear at present whether parathyroid hormone, analogues of parathyroid hormone-related peptide or insulin-like growth factor-1 will ever be available for routine clinical use. Increased understanding of the mechanisms of osteoclast recruitment and bone resorption has created a number of putative drug targets, but whether such agents will be economically viable competitors for the bisphosphonates, which are very inexpensive to manufacture, remains to be seen. The major challenge to those developing agents for use in osteoporosis is to find something that will stimulate growth of new bone and yet have an acceptable adverse effect profile. There are some promising candidates in this regard, based on animal studies, including the amylin-adrenomedullin family of peptides[105] and HMG-CoA reductase inhibitors,[106] but much remains to be done before their clinical potential can be judged.

13. Conclusions

There has been enormous progress in the pharmacological management of osteoporosis in the last two decades, resulting in a transition from therapeutic nihilism to a situation in which patients have real treatment options. Work needs to be done to further evaluate combination therapies. However, most of the available agents act by inhibiting bone resorption, so the principal challenge is to develop an effective bone anabolic agent with an acceptable safety profile.

References

1. Kameda T, Mano H, Yuasa T, et al. Estrogen inhibits bone resorption by directly inducing apoptosis of the bone-resorbing osteoclasts. J Exp Med 1997; 186: 489-95
2. Reid IR. Menopause. In: Favus MJ, editor. Primer on metabolic bone diseases and disorders of calcium metabolism. Washington, DC: ASBMR, 1999
3. Hofbauer LC, Khosla S, Dunstan CR, et al. Estrogen stimulates production of the anti-resorptive cytokine receptor osteoprotegerin in human osteoblastic cells. Bone 1998; 23 Suppl.: S172
4. Kanis JA, Melton LJ, Christiansen C, et al. Perspective: the diagnosis of osteoporosis. J Bone Miner Res 1994; 9: 1137-41
5. Tinetti ME, Baker DI, McAvay G, et al. A multifactorial intervention to reduce the risk of falling among elderly people living in the community. N Engl J Med 1994; 331: 821-7
6. Province MA, Hadley EC, Hornbrook MC, et al. The effects of exercise on falls in elderly patients: a preplanned meta-analysis of the FICSIT trials. JAMA 1995; 273: 1341-7
7. Lauritzen JB, Petersen MM, Lund B. Effect of external hip protectors on hip fractures. Lancet 1993; 341: 11-3
8. Eastell R. Treatment of postmenopausal osteoporosis. N Engl J Med 1998; 338: 736-46
9. Reid IR. The roles of calcium and vitamin D in the prevention of osteoporosis. Endocrinol Metab Clin North Am 1998; 27 (2): 389-98

10. Recker RR, Hinders S, Davies KM, et al. Correcting calcium nutritional deficiency prevents spine fractures in elderly women. J Bone Miner Res 1996; 11: 1961-6
11. Devine A, Dick IM, Heal SJ, et al. A 4-year follow-up study of the effects of calcium supplementation on bone density in elderly postmenopausal women. Osteoporos Int 1997; 7: 23-8
12. Riggs BL, Ofallon WM, Muhs J, et al. Long-term effects of calcium supplementation on serum parathyroid hormone level, bone turnover, and bone loss in elderly women. J Bone Miner Res 1998; 13: 168-74
13. Dawson-Hughes B, Dallal GE, Krall EA, et al. A controlled trial of the effect of calcium supplementation on bone density in postmenopausal women. N Engl J Med 1990; 323: 878-83
14. Elders PJ, Netelenbos JC, Lips P, et al. Calcium supplementation reduces vertebral bone loss in perimenopausal women: a controlled trial in 248 women between 46 and 55 years of age. J Clin Endocrinol Metab 1991; 73: 533-40
15. Reid IR, Ames RW, Evans MC, et al. Effect of calcium supplementation on bone loss in postmenopausal women. N Engl J Med 1993; 328: 460-4
16. Reid IR, Ames RW, Evans MC, et al. Long-term effects of calcium supplementation on bone loss and fractures in postmenopausal women: a randomized controlled trial. Am J Med 1995; 98: 331-5
17. Reid IR, Schooler BA, Hannon S, et al. The acute biochemical effects of four proprietary calcium supplements. Aust N Z J Med 1986; 16: 193-7
18. Chevalley T, Rizzoli R, Nydegger V, et al. Effects of calcium supplements on femoral bone mineral density and vertebral fracture rate in vitamin-D-replete elderly patients. Osteoporos Int 1994; 4: 245-52
19. Nieves JW, Komar L, Cosman F, et al. Calcium potentiates the effect of estrogen and calcitonin on bone mass: review and analysis. Am J Clin Nutr 1998; 67: 18-24
20. Ettinger B, Genant HK, Cann CE. Postmenopausal bone loss is prevented by treatment with low-dosage estrogen with calcium. Ann Intern Med 1987; 106: 40-5
21. Davis JW, Ross PD, Johnson NE, et al. Estrogen and calcium supplement use among Japanese-American women: effects upon bone loss when used singly and in combination. Bone 1995; 17: 369-73
22. Curhan GC, Willett WC, Speizer FE, et al. Comparison of dietary calcium with supplemental calcium and other nutrients as factors affecting the risk for kidney stones in women. Ann Intern Med 1997; 126 (7): 497-504
23. Malabanan A, Veronikis IE, Holick MF. Redefining vitamin D insufficiency. Lancet 1998; 351: 805-6
24. Ooms ME, Roos JC, Bezemer PD, et al. Prevention of bone loss by vitamin D supplementation in elderly women: a randomized double-blind trial. J Clin Endocrinol Metab 1995; 80: 1052-8
25. Dawson-Hughes B, Harris SS, Krall EA, et al. Rates of bone loss in postmenopausal women randomly assigned to one of two dosages of vitamin D. Am J Clin Nutr 1995; 61: 1140-5
26. Lips P, Graafmans WC, Ooms ME, et al. Vitamin D supplementation and fracture incidence in elderly persons: a randomized, placebo-controlled clinical trial. Ann Intern Med 1996; 124: 400-6
27. Heikinheimo RJ, Inkovaara JA, Harju EJ, et al. Annual injection of vitamin D and fractures of aged bones. Calcif Tissue Int 1992; 51: 105-10
28. Chapuy MC, Arlot ME, Duboeuf F, et al. Vitamin-D3 and calcium to prevent hip fractures in elderly women. N Engl J Med 1992; 327: 1637-42
29. Chapuy MC, Arlot ME, Delmas PD, et al. Effect of calcium and cholecalciferol treatment for three years on hip fractures in elderly women. BMJ 1994; 308: 1081-2
30. Dawson-Hughes B, Harris SS, Krall EA, et al. Effect of calcium and vitamin D supplementation on bone, density in men and women 65 years of age or older. N Engl J Med 1997; 337: 670-6
31. Komulainen M, Tuppurainen MT, Kroger H, et al. Vitamin D and HRT - no benefit additional to that of HRT alone in prevention of bone loss in early postmenopausal women: a 2.5-year randomized placebo-controlled study. Osteoporos Int 1997; 7: 126-32
32. Christiansen C, Christensen MS, McNair P, et al. Prevention of early postmenopausal bone loss: controlled 2-year study in 315 normal females. Eur J Clin Invest 1980; 10: 273-9
33. Nordin BEC, Horsman A, Crilly RG, et al. Treatment of spinal osteoporosis in postmenopausal women. BMJ 1980; 1: 451-4
34. Lindsay R, Hart DM, Forrest C, et al. Prevention of spinal osteoporosis in oophorectomised women. Lancet 1980; II: 1151-3
35. Lindsay R. Prevention and treatment of osteoporosis with ovarian hormones. Ann Chir Gynaecol 1988; 77: 219-23
36. Hosking D, Chilvers CED, Christiansen C, et al. Prevention of bone loss with alendronate in postmenopausal women under 60 years of age. N Engl J Med 1998; 338: 485-92
37. Bush TL, Wells HB, James MK, et al. Effects of hormone therapy on bone mineral density: results from the postmenopausal estrogen/progestin interventions (PEPI) trial. JAMA 1996; 276: 1389-96
38. Jensen GF, Christiansen C, Transbol I. Treatment of post menopausal osteoporosis: a controlled therapeutic trial comparing oestrogen/gestagen, 1,25-dihydroxy-vitamin D3 and calcium. Clin Endocrinol 1982; 16: 515-24
39. Lufkin EG, Wahner HW, O'Fallon WM, et al. Treatment of postmenopausal osteoporosis with transdermal estrogen. Ann Intern Med 1992; 117: 1-9
40. Lufkin EG, Riggs BL. Three-year follow-up on effects of transdermal estrogen [letter]. Ann Intern Med 1996; 125 (1): 77
41. Grey AB, Cundy TF, Reid IR. Continuous combined oestrogen/ progestin therapy is well tolerated and increases bone density at the hip and spine in post-menopausal osteoporosis. Clin Endocrinol 1994; 40: 671-7
42. Cauley JA, Seeley DG, Ensrud K, et al. Estrogen replacement therapy and fractures in older women. Ann Intern Med 1995; 122: 9-16
43. Michaelsson K, Baron JA, Farahmand BY, et al. Hormone replacement therapy and risk of hip fracture: population based case-control study. BMJ 1998; 316: 1858-63

44. Lafferty FW, Fiske ME. Postmenopausal estrogen replacement: a long-term cohort study. Am J Med 1994; 97: 66-77
45. Naessen T, Persson I, Thor L, et al. Maintained bone density at advanced ages after long term treatment with low dose oestradiol implants. Br J Obstet Gynaecol 1993; 100: 454-9
46. Christiansen C, Christensen MS, Transbol I. Bone mass in postmenopausal women after withdrawal of oestrogen/ gestagen replacement therapy. Lancet 1981; I: 459-61
47. Felson DT, Zhang YQ, Hannan MT, et al. The effect of postmenopausal estrogen therapy on bone density in elderly women. N Engl J Med 1993; 329: 1141-6
48. Schneider DL, Barrett-Connor EL, Morton DJ. Timing of postmenopausal estrogen for optimal bone mineral density: the Rancho Bernardo study. JAMA 1997; 277: 543-7
49. Grey A, Cundy T, Evans M, et al. Medroxyprogesterone acetate enhances the spinal bone mineral density response to oestrogen in late post-menopausal women. Clin Endocrinol 1996; 44: 293-6
50. Speroff L, Rowan J, Symons J, et al. The comparative effect on bone density, endometrium, and lipids of continuous hormones as replacement therapy (CHART Study): a randomized controlled trial. JAMA 1996; 276: 1397-403
51. Bjarnason NH, Bjarnason K, Haarbo J, et al. Tibolone: prevention of bone loss in late postmenopausal women. J Clin Endocrinol Metab 1996; 81: 2419-22
52. Wimalawansa SJ. Combined therapy with estrogen and etidronate has an additive effect on bone mineral density in the hip and vertebrae: four-year randomized study. Am J Med 1995; 99: 36-42
53. Wimalawansa SJ. A four-year randomized controlled trial of hormone replacement and bisphosphonate, alone or in combination, in women with postmenopausal osteoporosis. Am J Med 1998; 104: 219-26
54. Lindsay R, Cosman F, Cary DJ, et al. Effect of alendronate added to ongoing hormone replacement therapy on the bone mineral density of women with postmenopausal osteoporosis. Bone 1998; 23 Suppl.: S597
55. Gutteridge DH, Holzherr M, Will R, et al. Postmenopausal vertebral fractures: advantage of HRT plus calcitriol, over HRT alone, at total body and hip in malabsorbers and normal absorbers of Ca. Bone 1998; 23 Suppl.: S527
56. Alexandersen P, Hassager C, Sandholdt I, et al. Synergistic effect of hormone replacement therapy combined with monofluorophosphate on bone mass in late postmenopausal women. J Bone Miner Res 1997; 12 Suppl. 1: S104
57. Barrettconnor E, Grady D. Hormone replacement therapy, heart disease, and other considerations. Annu Rev Public Health 1998; 19: 55-72
58. Hulley S, Grady D, Bush T, et al. Randomized trial of estrogen plus progestin for secondary prevention of coronary heart disease in postmenopausal women. JAMA 1998; 280: 605-13
59. Beral V, Bull D, Doll R, et al. Breast cancer and hormone replacement therapy: collaborative reanalysis of data from 51 epidemiological studies of 52,705 women with breast cancer and 108,411 women without breast cancer. Lancet 1997; 350: 1047-59
60. Love RR, Mazess RB, Barden HS, et al. Effects of tamoxifen on bone mineral content in postmenopausal women with breast cancer. N Engl J Med 1991; 326: 852-6
61. Grey AB, Stapleton JP, Evans MC, et al. The effect of the anti-estrogen tamoxifen on cardiovascular risk factors in normal postmenopausal women. J Clin Endocrinol Metab 1995; 80: 3191-5
62. Grey AB, Stapleton JP, Evans MC, et al. The effect of the antiestrogen tamoxifen on bone mineral density in normal late postmenopausal women. Am J Med 1995; 99: 636-41
63. Delmas PD, Bjarnason NH, Mitlak BH, et al. Effects of raloxifene on bone mineral density, serum cholesterol concentrations, and uterine endometrium in postmenopausal women. N Engl J Med 1997; 337: 1641-7
64. Lufkin EG, Whitaker MD, Nickelsen T, et al. Treatment of established postmenopausal osteoporosis with raloxifene: a randomized. J Bone Miner Res 1998; 13: 1747-54
65. Ettinger B, Black DM, Mitlak BH, et al. Reduction in vertebral fracture risk in postmenopausal women with osteoporosis treated with raloxifene. JAMA 1999; 282: 637-45
66. Cummings SR, Eckert S, Krueger KA, et al. The effect of raloxifene on risk of breast cancer in postmenopausal women: results from the MORE randomized trial. JAMA 1999; 281: 2189-97
67. Luckman SP, Hughes DE, Coxon FP, et al. Nitrogen-containing bisphosphonates inhibit the mevalonate pathway and prevent post-translational prenylation of gtp-binding proteins, including ras. J Bone Miner Res 1998; 13: 581-9
68. Ebetino FH, Francis MD, Rogers MJ, et al. Mechanisms of action of etidronate and other bisphosphonates. Rev Cont Pharmacother 1998; 9: 233-43
69. Reid IR, King AR, Alexander CJ, et al. Prevention of steroid-induced osteoporosis with (3-amino-1-hydroxypropylidene)-1,1-bisphosphonate (APD). Lancet 1988; I: 143-6
70. Storm T, Thamsborg G, Steiniche T, et al. Effect of intermittent cyclical etidronate therapy on bone mass and fracture rate in postmenopausal osteoporosis. N Engl J Med 1990; 322: 1265-71
71. Watts NB, Harris ST, Genant HK, et al. Intermittent cyclical etidronate treatment of postmenopausal osteoporosis. N Engl J Med 1990; 323: 73-9
72. Liberman UA, Weiss SR, Broll J, et al. Effect of oral alendronate on bone mineral density and the incidence of fractures in postmenopausal osteoporosis. N Engl J Med 1995; 333: 1437-43
73. Black DM, Cummings SR, Karpf DB, et al. Randomised trial of effect of alendronate on risk of fracture in women with existing vertebral fractures. Lancet 1996; 348: 1535-41
74. Chavassieux PM, Arlot ME, Reda C, et al. Histomorphometric assessment of the long-term effects of alendronate on bone quality and remodeling in patients with osteoporosis. J Clin Invest 1997; 100: 1475-80
75. Lufkin EG, Argueta R, Whitaker MD, et al. Pamidronate: an unrecognized problem in gastrointestinal tolerability. Osteoporos Int 1994; 4: 320-2
76. Degroen PC, Lubbe DF, Hirsch LJ, et al. Esophagitis associated with the use of alendronate. N Engl J Med 1996; 335: 1016-21

77. Graham DY, Malaty HM, Goodgame R. Primary amino-bisphosphonates: a new class of gastrotoxic drugs - comparison of alendronate and aspirin. Am J Gastroenterol 1997; 92: 1322-5
78. Mackay FJ, Wilton LV, Pearce GL, et al. United Kingdom experience with alendronate and oesophageal reactions. Br J Gen Pract 1998; 48: 1161-2
79. Jones G, Nguyen T, Sambrook PN, et al. Thiazide diuretics and fractures: can meta-analysis help? J Bone Miner Res 1995; 10: 106-11
80. LaCroix Z, Ott SM, Ichikawa LE, et al. Low dose thiazide prevents bone loss in older adults: results of a 3-year randomized, double-blind controlled trial. Bone 1998; 23 Suppl.: S151
81. Reid IR, Ames RW, Orr-Walker BJ, et al. Hydrochlorothiazide reduces loss of cortical bone in normal postmenopausal women: a randomized controlled trial. Bone 1998; 23 Suppl.: S584
82. Christiansen C, Christensen MS, Rodbro P, et al. Effect of 1,25-dihydroxy-vitamin D3 in itself or combined with hormone treatment in preventing postmenopausal osteoporosis. Eur J Clin Invest 1981; 11: 305-9
83. Jensen GF, Meinecke B, Boesen J, et al. Does 1,25(OH)2 D3 accelerate spinal bone loss? Clin Orthop 1985; 192: 215-21
84. Falch JA, Odegaard OR, Finnanger M, et al. Postmenopausal osteoporosis: no effect of three years treatment with 1,25-dihydroxycholecalciferol. Acta Med Scand 1987; 221: 199-204
85. Ott SM, Chesnut CH. Calcitriol treatment is not effective in postmenopausal osteoporosis. Ann Intern Med 1989; 110: 267-74
86. Gallagher JC, Goldgar D. Treatment of postmenopausal osteoporosis with high doses of synthetic calcitriol: a randomized controlled study. Ann Intern Med 1990; 113: 649-55
87. Aloia JF, Vaswani A, Yeh JK, et al. Calcitriol in the treatment of postmenopausal osteoporosis. Am J Med 1988; 84: 401-8
88. Tilyard MW, Spears GF, Thomson J, et al. Treatment of postmenopausal osteoporosis with calcitriol or calcium. N Engl J Med 1992; 326: 357-62
89. Reid IR. Vitamin D and its metabolites in the management of osteoporosis. In: Marcus R, Feldman D, Kelsey J, editors. Osteoporosis. San Diego (CA): Academic Press, 1996
90. Luisetto G, Bottega F, Zangari M, et al. Effects of three therapeutic regimens on postmenopausal bone loss in oophorectomized women. Curr Ther Res Clin Exp 1996; 57: 839-48
91. Itoi H, Minakami H, Sato I. Comparison of the long-term effects of oral estriol with the effects of conjugated estrogen, 1-alpha- hydroxyvitamin d-3 and calcium lactate on vertebral bone loss in early menopausal women. Maturitas 1997; 28: 11-7
92. Frediani B, Allegri A, Bisogno S, et al. Effects of combined treatment with calcitriol plus alendronate on bone mass and bone turnover in postmenopausal osteoporosis two years of continuous treatment. Clin Drug Invest 1998; 15: 235-44
93. Masud T, Mulcahy B, Thompson AV, et al. Effects of cyclical etidronate combined with calcitriol versus cyclical etidronate alone on spine and femoral neck bone mineral density in postmenopausal osteoporotic women. Ann Rheum Dis 1998; 57: 346-9
94. Eddy DM, Johnston CC, Cummings SR, et al. Osteoporosis: review of the evidence for prevention, diagnosis, and treatment and cost-effectiveness analysis. Osteoporos Int 1998; 8 Suppl. 4: 1-88
95. Arnala I, Saastamoinen J, Alhava EM. Salmon calcitonin in the prevention of bone loss at perimenopause. Bone 1996; 18: 629-32
96. Stock JL, Avioli LV, Baylink DJ, et al. Calcitonin-salmon nasal spray reduces the incidence of new vertebral fractures in postmenopausal women: three year interim results of the PROOF study. J Bone Miner Res 1997; 12 Suppl. 1: S149
97. Silverman SL, Chesnut C, Andriano K, et al. Salmon calcitonin nasal spray (NS-CT) reduces risk of vertebral fracture(s) (VF) in established osteoporosis and has continuous efficacy with prolonged treatment: accrued 5 year worldwide data of the PROOF study. Bone 1998; 23 Suppl.: S174
98. Riggs BL, Hodgson SF, O'Fallon WM, et al. Effect of fluoride treatment on the fracture rate in postmenopausal women with osteoporosis. N Engl J Med 1990; 322: 802-9
99. Caverzasio J, Imai T, Ammann P, et al. Aluminum potentiates the effect of fluoride on tyrosine phosphorylation and osteoblast replication in vitro and bone mass in vivo. J Bone Miner Res 1996; 11: 46-55
100. Meunier PJ, Sebert JL, Reginster JY, et al. Fluoride salts are no better at preventing new vertebral fractures than calcium-vitamin D in postmenopausal osteoporosis: the Favos study. Osteoporos Int 1998; 8: 4-12
101. Pak CYC, Sakhaee K, Adamshuet B, et al. Treatment of postmenopausal osteoporosis with slow-release sodium fluoride: final report of a randomized controlled trial. Ann Intern Med 1995; 123: 401-8
102. Reginster JY, Meurmans L, Zegels B, et al. The effect of sodium monofluorophosphate plus calcium on vertebral fracture rate in postmenopausal women with moderate osteoporosis: a randomized, controlled trial. Ann Intern Med 1998; 129 (1): 1-8
103. Need AG, Horowitz M, Bridges A, et al. Effects of nandrolone decanoate and antiresorptive therapy on vertebral density in osteoporotic postmenopausal women. Arch Int Med 1989; 149: 57-60
104. Reid IR, Wattie DJ, Evans MC, et al. Continuous therapy with pamidronate, a potent bisphosphonate, in postmenopausal osteoporosis. J Clin Endocrinol Metab 1994; 79: 1595-9
105. Cornish J, Callon KE, King AR, et al. Systemic administration of amylin increases bone mass, linear growth, and adiposity in adult male mice. Am J Physiol 1998; 38: E694-9
106. Mundy G, Gutteriez G, Garrett R, et al. Identification of a new class of powerful stimulators of new bone formation in vivo, clarification of mechanism of action, and use in animal models of osteoporosis. Bone 1998; 23 Suppl.: S183

Correspondence: Dr *Ian R. Reid*, Department of Medicine, University of Auckland, Private Bag 92019, Auckland, New Zealand.
E-mail: i.reid@auckland.ac.nz

Osteoporosis in Men

New Insights into Aetiology, Pathogenesis, Prevention and Management

Peter Robert Ebeling

Department of Diabetes and Endocrinology, The Royal Melbourne Hospital, Melbourne, Victoria, Australia

Osteoporosis is increasingly being recognised in men.[1] In the next 20 years it is likely to emerge as an important public health problem both in the West and in the developing world, as numbers of elderly men increase and the age-specific incidence of hip fractures in men also increases. It is projected that, over the next 15 years, ≈30% of hip fractures will occur in men.[2] Recent epidemiological data show the incidence of vertebral fractures in men to be 0.73 per 1000 person-years, which is half the incidence seen in women,[3] but is not 10%, as previously reported.[4] However, even this is likely to be a conservative estimate because only ≈30% of vertebral fractures are symptomatic and come to clinical attention.

Recent data show that vertebral fracture rates are as great in men as in women but, because women live longer, the lifetime risk of a vertebral fracture from age 50 onward is 16% in White women and only 5% in White men.[5] In Australian men aged 60 years, the lifetime risk of an osteoporotic fracture is 29%, about half that in women. In men aged 60 to 80 years, these will be predominantly non-hip fractures.[6] Depending on age, between 60 and 90% of hip and vertebral fractures in White men aged >45 years can be attributed to osteoporosis.[7]

It is also important to recognise that there is likely to be increased morbidity and mortality following hip fractures in men compared with women.[8] One month after hip fracture, the mortality rate in men was 16%. 55% of men with hip fractures were discharged to nursing homes. Only 41% of survivors recovered their prefracture level of functioning. Age and deterioration in postoperative mental state increased the risk of early death. The prevalence of both moderate and severe vertebral deformities increases with age in men and severe vertebral deformities are associated with a greater functional impairment in men than in women.[9]

Cost estimates for these fragility fractures in Australian men range between $AU70 to 230 million per year.[4,10] Geographical variation in fracture rates also occurs in men; their hip fracture risk is higher than that of women in Beijing and fracture rates for men in some parts of the US and Europe continue to increase while those for women have increased in developing countries such as Singapore.[6] Thus, osteoporosis in men is already a public health problem and its economic and personal burden will increase unless public health strategies are initiated to prevent the disease or effective therapeutic options for established disease are identified.

In the past, the problem of osteoporosis in women has overshadowed research into osteoporosis in men, so little is known of the factors causing low bone mass or increased bone loss in men. Although few prospective studies of fragility fractures in men have been made, low bone mass, risk factors for falling and other factors important in the aetiology of fractures in women are likely to be associated with fragility fractures in men.

A recent prospective study has shown that men and women have the same risk of vertebral fracture for the same absolute calcaneal bone mass;[11] however, it is uncertain if the same relationships exist for spinal and proximal femur bone mineral density (BMD). The Dubbo Epidemiology Study demonstrated that increased body sway and decreased quadriceps strength in addition to low femoral neck BMD were associated with an increased risk of hip fractures in men.[12] In a large case-control study from Rochester, conditions linked with an increased risk of falling were also associated with a 7-fold increase in hip fracture risk, while diseases linked with secondary osteoporosis doubled the fracture risk.[13] Overall, these factors accounted for ≈72% of hip fractures in men. In a smaller case-control study that examined risk factors including serum free testosterone levels, hypogonadism was associated with a 4.6-fold increase in hip fracture rates after adjusting for race.[14] In men with rheumatoid arthritis, the risk of hip fracture was doubled; corticosteroid use also independently increased hip fracture risk by 2.6-fold.[15]

1. Bone Mass and Rates of Bone Loss in Men

Bone mass is thought to be largely genetically determined. Studies in twins have shown that genetic factors account for ≈60% of the variance in bone mass in both men and women.[16,17] Nevertheless, environmental factors also make an important contribution to bone mass. Greater muscle strength and physical activity are associated with greater bone mass in men.[18] Recent prospective studies of radial bone loss in older men show that cigarette smoking and moderate alcohol consumption contribute to bone loss, as they do in women.[19] Bone loss from the femoral neck occurred at a rate of 0.82% per year in men, a slightly lower rate than that in women.[20] No bone loss occurred at the spine; however, the rate of loss from the hip increased with aging. Overall, prospective studies of bone loss in men have been limited, partly because age-related bone loss occurs at a relatively slow rate and also because, given the precision of current methods for measuring bone mass, accurate estimates of rates of bone loss, particularly at the femoral neck, require long periods of follow-up.

Peak bone mass is greater in men than women (fig. 1) predominantly because they have larger bones.[22] This difference is possibly androgen-dependent. In tubular bones, total width is greater and cortical thickness is increased with reduced cortical porosity.[23] Vertebral cross-sectional area is 25% greater in men than women; this is due to an increase in vertebral width and depth (but not height). Age-related vertebral bone loss is less in men than in women because the vertebrae increase in cross-

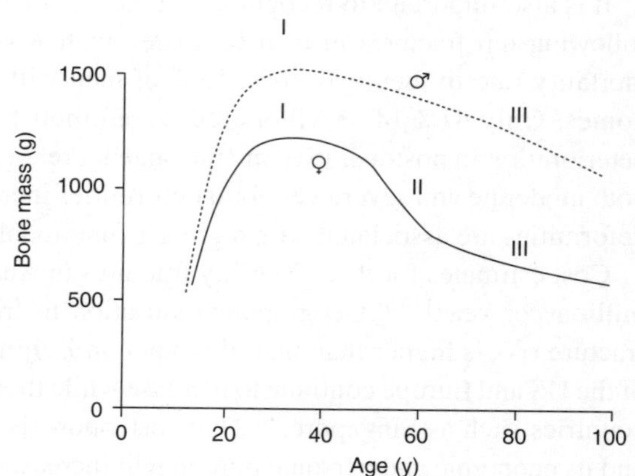

Fig. 1. Changes in bone mass with age in men and women (reproduced from Riggs & Melton,[21] with permission). **I** = peak bone mass; **II** = postmenopausal bone loss; **III** = age-related bone loss.

sectional area by 25 to 30% with aging in men as a result of subperiosteal apposition of new bone.[24] This also occurs in the long bones, with the girth of long bones increasing more in men than in women.[25] Hip axis length may also be different in men than in women, creating another anatomical advantage in reducing propensity to fracture.

Although age-related rates of bone loss at predominantly trabecular sites (distal radius, vertebrae and calcaneus) are similar in men and women, the pattern of loss is not. In men this is the result of generalised trabecular thinning, but in women there is a more marked loss of trabecular elements.[24]

2. Osteoporosis in Men

2.1 Possible Factors Affecting Age-Related Bone Loss

A number of explanations for excessive bone loss may coexist in the individual man with osteoporosis. Age-related bone loss alone can cause an increased risk of fracture. This may be related to a decline in bone formation with aging,[26,27] although some recent studies have also demonstrated an increase in bone turnover with aging in men.[28] However, newer bone resorption markers do not consistently increase with age.[29,30] In most studies of healthy men, higher levels of bone turnover markers have been associated with lower BMD of the proximal femur[27,28,30] and, less commonly, with lower spinal BMD.[27,29]

Changes in growth factors or cytokines may contribute to age-related bone loss, as do nutritional deficiencies, inactivity and loss of gonadal function. Dietary calcium deficiency is common in men, >50% of whom ingest less than the recommended daily allowance. Aging has also been associated with increased parathyroid hormone (PTH) levels,[31] decreased calcifediol (25-hydroxy vitamin D) levels[32] and, in some studies, decreased calcitriol (1,25-dihydroxy vitamin D_3) levels.[33,34] Intestinal resistance to calcitriol occurs in women with osteoporosis and it may also exist in men. This intestinal resistance may be receptor mediated or caused by post-receptor events.[35,36] There is growing evidence that the decrease in calcium absorption with aging in men is related to both reduced renal 1α-hydroxylase activity and reduced levels of calcitriol, as well as intestinal resistance to calcitriol. In this regard, active calcium absorption is reduced in men with spinal fractures.[36a] It is unlikely that the abnormal alleles of the vitamin D receptor (VDR) gene associated with low bone density[37] have a functional effect on reducing calcium absorption. Nevertheless, calcium supplementation has a greater effect on increasing bone density in women with the abnormal (BB) VDR allele.[38]

Although several reports have linked dietary calcium intake to bone density in men, the evidence is inconclusive. Some studies have found an effect of calcium intake on axial but not radial bone density.[39,40] Studies of relationships between calcium nutrition and hip fracture in men are suggestive of a beneficial effect but remain speculative.[41] A recent study examined the effects of dietary calcium supplementation on fragility fractures in non-institutionalised men and women aged >65 years. Men had only two fragility fractures in the placebo group. Rates of bone loss at the spine and femoral neck were reduced by ≈1% in the first year of calcium treatment, but not during the subsequent 2 years of the study, whereas total body bone loss was unaffected in the first year but reduced by a similar amount in the subsequent 2 years.[42]

Bodyweight and mechanical force have strong effects on bone density. Decreases in physical activity and muscle strength with aging may also contribute to age-related bone loss by reducing mechanical forces on skeletal tissues. Increases in serum leptin concentrations inhibit bone formation and reduce bone mass through a central hypothalamic relay. This process may interact with regulation of gonadal hormones.[42a] The relationship between changes in sex hormone levels with aging and age-related bone loss are discussed in more detail in section 3.

2.2 Secondary Pathological Causes of Osteoporosis

Thirty to 60% of men evaluated for vertebral fractures have another illness contributing to the presence of bone disease.[1] Glucocorticoid excess (predominantly exogenous) is the most common secondary cause, accounting for 16 to 18% of cases.[43] The pathophysiology of glucocorticoid-induced osteoporosis is similar in women and men and the most important mechanism is a direct inhibition of osteoblast activity and decreased osteoblast recruitment. However, muscle weakness, immobility, impaired intestinal calcium absorption, hypercalciuria and a reduction in serum testosterone levels also all contribute to glucocorticoid-associated bone loss.[44]

The link between alcohol (ethanol) abuse and bone diseases has been well established by epidemiological studies;[4] however, the mechanism of alcohol-related bone loss is unclear. Osteoblast function is decreased by alcohol as assessed by bone histomorphometric studies[45] and this also may be secondary to a direct toxic effect of alcohol on osteoblasts. Colecalciferol deficiency and reduced free serum testosterone concentrations in alcohol-induced bone disease may contribute to bone loss.[46]

Tobacco use is associated with decreased bone mass in women.[47] In a study in men, the relative risk of vertebral fracture in smokers was 2.3.[48] This risk was independent of alcohol consumption. The mechanism of this effect is unknown, but may relate to decreased bodyweight and decreased calcium absorption. However, another larger study did not support such a strong influence of tobacco on fracture risk.[12]

Gastrointestinal disease predisposes men to bone disease, as a result of intestinal malabsorption of calcium and colecalciferol. In particular, gastrectomy is a common association of vertebral osteoporosis in men. Other gastrointestinal diseases (coeliac disease, Crohn's disease, small intestinal resection) cause bone disease equally in men and women.[1] Hypercalciuria and nephrolithiasis in men are associated with osteopenia and this may be related to secondary hyperparathyroidism, increased calcitriol levels and increased bone turnover rates.

Anticonvulsant drug use (phenobarbital, phenytoin), thyrotoxicosis, immobilisation, liver and renal disease, multiple myeloma and systemic mastocytosis have all been associated with osteoporosis in both men and women.[1]

2.3 Idiopathic Osteoporosis

In ≈45% of men with symptomatic vertebral fractures, no known cause of bone disease could be identified.[49] The wide age range of men with idiopathic osteoporosis (23 to 86 years) suggests that in some men there may be a premature onset of age-related osteoporosis; however, the pathogenesis may differ in younger men. Importantly, the structural bone defect is similar to that in adult male hypogonadism with reduced trabecular numbers, rather than reduced trabecular thickness. Nevertheless, there are no consistent features of idiopathic osteoporosis in men. In one study, intestinal calcium absorption was reduced and calcitriol levels were decreased.[49] Calcium balance was also negative in 16 men with idiopathic osteoporosis because net calcium absorption was insufficient to offset urinary calcium losses.[49]

Although a defect in osteoblastic function has been identified in idiopathic male osteoporosis, it is not a consistent finding.[50-52] The age of the individual may be important in this regard, with young men having reduced histomorphometric indices of bone formation, while older men had similar bone formation rates to age-matched controls, but evidence of slightly increased bone resorption.[53] Unfortunately, there are no data concerning the levels of currently available biochemical bone markers in osteoporotic men. As in hypogonadism, the structural bone defect is a reduction in trabecular number rather than a decline in trabecular thickness; however trabecular connectivity has not been formally addressed in any study.

3. Sex Hormone Effects on Bone in Men

3.1 Androgen Effects

Although there is no abrupt cessation of testicular function or 'andropause' comparable with the menopause in women, both total and free testosterone concentrations decline with age in men. The age-related reduction in total testosterone is accompanied by a proportionately greater increase in sex hormone binding globulin, resulting in a larger decline in free testosterone with age in men.[54] Age-related decreases in adrenal androgens are greater than for testosterone and may have more impact on age-related bone loss.[55] A limited correlation exists between free testosterone levels with bone density at some, but not all, skeletal sites and these findings have been inconsistent between studies.[40]

One of the most common secondary causes of osteoporosis in men is hypogonadism. This is associated with a phase of rapid bone loss and increases in biochemical markers of bone turnover, as it is in women. This is followed by a phase of bone loss associated with low bone turnover. The role of androgens in bone accretion and skeletal maintenance in men has been poorly studied.

In addition, it is uncertain whether testosterone therapy of eugonadal men results in significant increases in bone density. One nonrandomised study of parenteral testosterone therapy of eugonadal men detected increases in spinal but not proximal femur bone mass.[56] However, a double blind, placebo-controlled trial of transdermal testosterone showed no effect.[57] Nevertheless, hypogonadism is present in as many as 30% of men with osteoporotic vertebral fracture,[1] and low testosterone concentrations are also common in men with hip fractures.

As previously noted, androgens are important in both attainment of peak bone mass and in the maintenance of bone mass in adult men. In prepubertal hypogonadism, the bone deficit is more marked in cortical compartments than that in adult-onset hypogonadism, where trabecular bone loss occurs with a reduction in trabecular numbers. Histomorphometric studies have also shown that bone formation rates are reduced in hypogonadism;[58] however, bone turnover increases acutely following orchidectomy.[59] Testosterone replacement in hypogonadal men increased spinal and distal radius BMD by ≈6% per year, although cortical deficits are not replaced.[60,61] Body fat and biochemical bone turnover markers decreased, while lean muscle mass increased with testosterone therapy.

In European hypogonadal males with fractures, calcitriol levels were decreased. Both bone formation parameters and plasma calcitriol levels increased following testosterone treatment.[50] In contrast, US studies have not demonstrated reduced bone formation rates, but a slight increase in mean remodelling rate comparable with postmenopausal estrogen deficiency in women.[58] Thus, nutritional colecalciferol deficiency may have contributed to the European study findings.

3.2 The Androgen Receptor as a Transcription Factor

Overall, there are relatively low concentrations of androgen and estrogen receptors in osteoblasts in men. Androgens and estrogens affect bone cells by indirect as well as direct mechanisms secondary to changes in concentrations of systemic and local factors. Several of these effects, including proliferation, growth factor and cytokine production, and bone matrix protein production (type I collagen, osteocalcin, osteopontin), are mediated by the androgen receptor (AR). The AR is a member of the steroid hormone/nuclear receptor superfamily. The AR is a ligand-dependent transcription factor, and comprises three functional domains: the steroid-binding domain, DNA-binding domain and amino-terminal domain.

The amino-terminal domain of the AR is involved in the modulation of transcription activation (transactivation).[62] Different transactivation regions within the amino-terminal domain of the AR may be active in regulating different genes, allowing cell-specific and gene-specific regulation of expression. Within the amino-terminal domain are two polymorphic regions: a stretch of glutamine (Gln) residues, encoded by CAG repeats, with the number of Glns normally varying between 11 and 31, and with most individuals having between 18 and 25 repeats;[63,64] and a stretch of GGN repeats that ranges in size between 16 and 24 Gly repeats.[65]

Studies on the AR suggest that the poly Gln stretch in the amino-terminal domain acts as a repressor of transcription activation. Deletion of the Gln repeats in the amino-terminal domain causes increased transactivation from androgen responsive promoters. Studies have shown that changes in the CAG/Gln length can alter transcription activation of AR responsive genes in a promoter-dependent manner.[66] However, these studies have been limited to investigating AR with either normal (n = 20) versus greatly increased or decreased numbers of CAG repeats.

3.3 Androgen-Responsive Genes

Androgen-responsive genes include the two androgen-dependent kallikrein-like genes, prostate specific antigen (PSA) and human glandular kallikrein 1. PSA can specifically cleave insulin-like growth factor binding protein-3 (IGFBP-3; somatomedin binding protein-3), increasing the amount of locally bioavailable insulin-like growth factor-1 (IGF-1; somatomedin-1).[67] Epidermal growth factor receptor expression and transforming growth factor-α (TGFα) secretion are upregulated by androgens.[68,69] Androgens may also directly reduce IGF-3 expression, suggesting that one target for androgenic regulation of cell growth may be through IGF-3 regulation.[70] Castration causes an increase in *c-myc* gene expression in the ventral rat prostate; an effect reversible by androgen treatment;[69] thus, *c-myc* may also mediate androgenic effects.

Type I collagen is a sex hormone-responsive protein produced during osteoblast proliferation. Type I procollagen propeptide (PICP) is a bone formation marker. Serum PICP levels decrease in men but increase in women with aging,[26] as well as increasing during IGF-1 treatment.[71] Low serum levels of IGF-1 have been reported in men with idiopathic osteoporosis and may thus be partly responsible for the low bone formation rates observed in some men with this condition.[72] A defect in the type I collagen gene has also been identified in a family with osteoporosis affecting both male and female members.[73] Recently, a polymorphism in the Sp1 transcriptional control region of the collagen type I α1 gene has been shown to be over-represented in postmenopausal osteoporotic women and associated with low BMD.[74] No studies of Sp1 polymorphisms or their relationship to AR alleles have been performed in men.

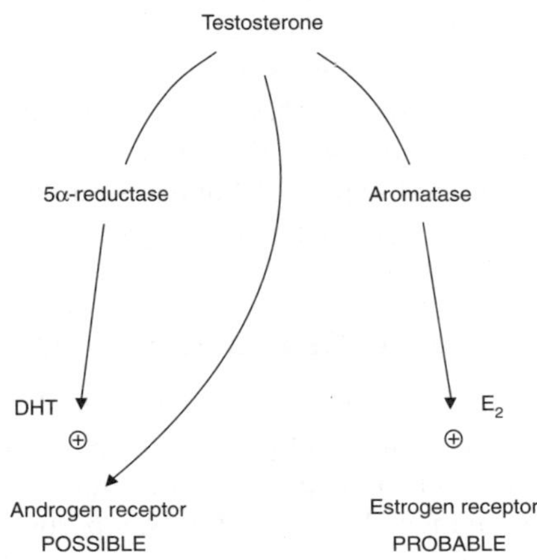

Fig. 2. Direct and indirect effects of androgens on skeletal maintenance (reproduced from Vanderscheueren et al.,[75] with permission). **DHT** = dihydrotestosterone; **E_2** = estradiol.

3.4 Estrogen Effects

There is increasing evidence that estrogens have an important role in skeletal maintenance in men as well as in women (fig. 2). Peripheral aromatisation of androgens to estrogens occurs in men as well as in women. In addition, osteoblast-like cells can aromatise androgens into estrogens. Aged male rats treated with an aromatase inhibitor had similar bone loss to orchidectomised rats, indicating aromatisation of androgens into estrogen may partially explain the effects of androgens on bone.[75] Human models also exist for the effects of estrogens on the skeleton. A man with a stop mutation in the estrogen receptor gene and high circulating estradiol levels had failure of epiphyseal fusion and continued skeletal growth and severe osteoporosis.[76] Similarly, an aromatase-deficient man developed tall stature and osteoporosis, and low-dose estrogen therapy resulted in a large increase in bone density.[77,78]

A recent study has shown that bone density at all skeletal sites was significantly positively associated with greater serum estradiol levels in men aged >65 years.[79] There were also negative associations between serum testosterone and bone density at the spine and hip, and sex-hormone binding globulin was negatively associated with bone density only at the greater trochanter. Bodyweight, age and serum sex steroids accounted for 30% of the variability of bone density in men with consistent positive associations between bone density and serum estradiol levels in men. Importantly, within the normal range, lower serum testosterone levels were not associated with low bone density in men.

In transsexual men treated with estrogens and antiandrogens, bone density increased, and both bone turnover and serum IGF-1 levels decreased. In contrast, testosterone administration to transsexual women increased bone formation, but this did not result in increased bone density, despite increases in serum IGF-1 levels.[80] Thus, adult bone remodelling may be preferentially regulated via the estrogen receptor (ER), with estrogen playing a pivotal role in skeletal mineralisation in both men and women. In support of this hypothesis, both male and female ER gene knockout mice have BMD that is 20 to 25% lower than wild-type mice.[81] The latter experiment has been difficult to interpret because of the smaller skeletons of the ER gene knockout mice compared with wild type mice. Nevertheless, less severe ER defects could also be responsible for idiopathic osteoporosis in some men.

Recently, *Pvu*II and *Xba*I restriction length polymorphisms of the ER gene have been associated with low bone density in healthy postmenopausal Japanese women.[82] Women with the Px haplotype had lumbar spine and total body BMD 0.47 and 0.64 SDs lower, respectively, than Px haplotype-negative women. No studies of this ER haplotype have been performed in men.

4. Treatment of Osteoporosis in Men

There has been one study of specific drug therapy for osteoporosis in men with fragility fractures as a primary end-point.[82a] There have been two randomised placebo-controlled trials and few uncontrolled prospective trials of therapies for osteoporosis using BMD as an end-point in men. Therapies for osteoporosis can either inhibit bone resorption (bone density initially increases with infilling of the remodelling space and then remains stable) or stimulate new bone formation (fig. 3). A summary of studies that have examined drug efficacy in men with osteoporosis is shown in table I.

To summarise these limited studies: intermittent low-dose sodium monofluorophosphate and calcium reduced vertebral fractures and increased spine and hip BMDs in men with idiopathic osteoporosis.[82a] Alendronate treatment of men with idiopathic osteoporosis or hypogonadism-related osteoporosis has recently been shown to increase spinal and hip BMD; there was also a nonsignificant trend for a reduction in vertebral fractures.[88b] Calcitonin resulted in increases in total body calcium but was not different to calcium and/or cholecalciferol supplements in this regard.[83] It also reduced biochemical markers of bone turnover in the short-term in castrated men, although effects on bone density were not studied.[59]

Cyclical etidronic acid (disodium etidronate) given in two dosage regimens caused increased lumbar spine bone density at 2 years; however, bone density at both the distal and proximal radius decreased over the same time, while proximal femur bone density remained unchanged.[84] This study was uncontrolled, so it is not known whether changes occurring with etidronic acid were different from those expected with placebo or calcium alone. In 42 men with vertebral crush fractures, treated with 3-monthly cycles of disodium etidronate for over 2 years, spinal BMD increased by 3.2% per year and proximal femur BMD did not change.[85] In a small retrospective study of 10 men with osteoporosis treated with cyclical etidronic acid, the increase in spinal BMD was greater being 9.0% at 1 year.[86]

Testosterone treatment of eugonadal men with vertebral crush fractures for 6 months increased spinal BMD by 5%. During treatment, free androgen and estradiol levels increased by 90 and 45%, respectively,[87] and bone turnover markers decreased. The change in spinal BMD was correlated with the change in estradiol but not testosterone, suggesting that estrogen may decrease bone turnover

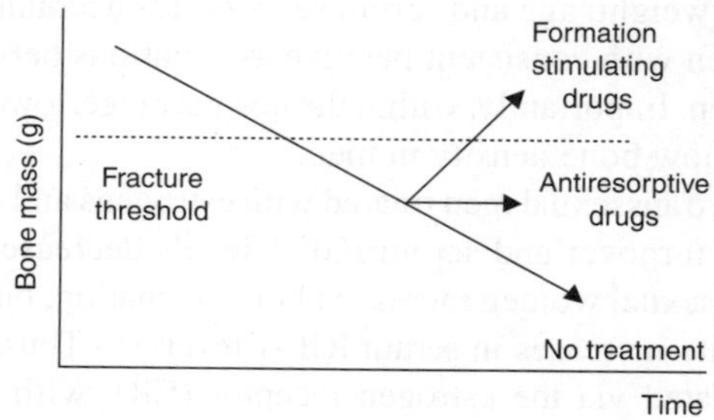

Fig. 3. Effect of treatment on bone mass.

Table I. Studies examining drug efficacy in men with osteoporosis

Agent	Osteoporosis type	Duration	No. of patients	Primary end-point(s)	Control group(s)	Effect	Ref.
Intermittent sodium monofluorophosphate + calcium	Idiopathic	3 years	64	LS BMD Hip BMD Vertebral fractures	Calcium	+ + +	82a
Calcitriol	Idiopathic	2 years	41	LS BMD FN BMD TB BMC	Calcium	0 0 0	88a
Alendronate	Idiopathic Hypogonadism	2 years	241	LS BMD Hip BMD	Calcium, colecalciferol	+	88b
Calcitonin	Idiopathic	2 years	8	TB BMC	Calcium, colecalciferol	+	83
				Radius BMC	Colecalciferol	0	
	Hypogonadal	3 months	9	BBM	Crossover (self control)	+	59
Etidronic acid	Mixed	2 years	36	LS BMD FN BMD DR BMC PR BMC	Nil	+ 0 – –	84
	Vertebral fractures	2 years	42	LS BMD FN BMD	Nil	+ 0	85
	Idiopathic secondary	1 year	10	LS BMD FN BMD	Nil	+ 0	86
Testosterone esters	Vertebral fractures	6 months	21	LS BMD FN BMD BBM	Nil	+ 0 +	87
Parathyroid hormone and calcitriol (1,25-dihydroxy vitamin D_3)	Idiopathic	1 year	8	Trabecular BMD DR BMC	Nil	+ 0	88

BBM = biochemical bone markers; **BMC** = bone mineral content; **BMD** = bone mineral density; **DR** = distal radius; **FN** = proximal femur; **LS** = lumbar spine; **PR** = proximal radius; **TB** = trabecular bone; + = a positive effect of active treatment; **0** = no effect of active treatment; **–** = no effect.

more effectively than testosterone in men.

Combined with human PTH injections, calcitriol increased trabecular bone density in middle-aged men with idiopathic osteoporosis.[88] Although it is not known whether similar effects would be seen with either PTH or calcitriol treatment alone, in view of recent studies in postmenopausal women with osteoporosis treated with PTH, it is likely that this hormone was primarily responsible for the increase in BMD. Our recent small double-blind, double-placebo study of calcitriol 0.5 mg/day or calcium 1000 mg/day in men with idiopathic osteoporosis showed no difference in effects on spinal or femoral neck BMD or total body BMC over 2 years.[88a]

5. Future Options

5.1 Estrogen And Specific Estrogen Receptor-Modulating Drugs (SERMs)

Because estrogen concentrations are important determinants of BMD in men, it is possible that low-dose estrogen therapy might increase BMD in men as well as in women. However, it is unlikely that the majority of men would accept the adverse effects related to estrogen therapy.

Of particular concern is the potential for adverse cardiovascular effects in men. While specific estrogen receptor modulating drugs (SERMs) would avoid adverse effects on libido, it is uncertain whether some or all of these drugs would prevent potential cardiovascular adverse effects such as thromboembolism. Because rates of bone loss are low in men, clinical trials of SERMs in men would need to be of at least 3 years' duration and cardiovascular end-points would also need to be carefully examined in any such study, particularly effects on LDL cholesterol.

5.2 Bone Formation–Stimulating Drugs

5.2.1 Parathyroid Hormone Peptides

As early as 1929, Fuller Albright showed that PTH extract could increase bone density in the rat. These findings have been difficult to translate to the treatment of osteoporosis in humans because of the expense and injectable nature of the peptides, and also because of important species differences in bone and mineral metabolism.

Two controlled studies of teriperatide (hPTH-1-34) and hPTH-1-38 given for 3 years or 1 year, respectively, have examined changes in bone mass in postmenopausal women receiving concurrent hormone replacement therapy.[89,90] Lumbar spine bone mineral content (BMC), that is, bone mass not adjusted for bone area or volume, increased by 11% over 2 years and this increase was maintained following cessation of PTH therapy, albeit after a small but rapid decrease of 2% in bone mass. Total body bone mass increased by 6% while femoral neck BMD decreased by 3.2% over 3 years in both groups. No changes in spinal or total body mass occurred in the control group.

An elegant study of histomorphometric bone turnover indices during PTH therapy has shown that bone formation was initiated on surfaces that would not have had time to be fully excavated by osteoclasts.[91] Later biopsies demonstrated increased wall thickness of completed newborn packets, moderate rather than large increases in bone formation indices and modest changes in bone resorption indices. Enhanced trabecular connectivity as well as increased trabecular thickness may have been responsible for the increased bone volume. An interesting finding in postmenopausal women treated for 1 year with alendronic acid is that nocturnal increases in PTH are associated with decreases in bone turnover and increases in bone density.[92] PTH also prevents bone loss associated with medical oophorectomy for the treatment of endometriosis.[93] PTH combined with calcitriol increases trabecular bone mass in men, as noted in section 4.[88]

As PTH shares the PTH-1 receptor with parathyroid hormone-related protein (PTHrP), it is likely that PTHrP (1-34) analogues will have similar effects on bone to PTH. Such analogues are anabolic for bone in primate models of osteoporosis and have undergone phase I and II clinical trials. However, it is not yet known whether the newly identified PTH-2 receptor contributes to the anabolic effects of PTH/PTHrP. PTHrP, in addition to IGF-1, transforming growth factor-β and prostaglandins may also act as a local modulator of PTH action.

Because of its expense and its injectable mode of administration, PTH cannot be currently regarded as a suitable first line treatment for osteoporosis. In the future, PTH peptides may be an effective first- or second-line treatment for osteoporosis, particularly in those patients in whom other treatment modalities such as bisphosphonates are perceived to have failed, or in those with very low bone density and presumed trabecular loss.

5.2.2 Growth Hormone and Insulin-Like Growth Factor

Both growth hormone (GH) and IGF-1 stimulate osteoblastic differentiation *in vitro*. In animal models, GH and IGF-1 enhance longitudinal growth, bone formation and bone mass; however, responses to GH or IGF-1 are not equivalent and depend on the species, the animal's GH status and the mode of administration. Although rhGH and IGF-1 both enhance trabecular and cortical bone density in GH-deficient patients, rhGH administration to healthy men or women results only in small, inconsistent changes in BMD.[94,95]

Growth hormone treatment of elderly men and women is also associated with a high incidence of unpleasant adverse effects (oedema, glucose intolerance and bilateral carpal tunnel syndrome). Both GH and IGF-1 stimulate bone turnover and activate remodelling osteons. The intriguing possibility exists that low dose IGF-1 may directly increase osteoblastic function with only a minimal decrease in bone resorption.[71,96] At these doses the adverse effects of higher dose IGF-1 (bloating, oedema, parotid discomfort, tachycardia, orthostatic hypotension) are avoided.[71]

Men with idiopathic osteoporosis have low circulating IGF-1 concentrations. Administration of IGF-1 to these men increases bone formation markers more than resorption markers. Studies of changes in BMD with IGF-1 treatment in osteoporotic men and women are currently underway. A new IGF-1 preparation combines the drug with IGF-3, prolonging the half-life of IGF-1. It has yet to be evaluated in humans. However, because there are no studies of the effects of IGF-1 on bone mass or of the effects of either rhGH or IGF-1 on fracture rates, the results of longer-term clinical trials in men are required before the safety of these agents can be assessed.

6. Effects of Treatment on Healthy Men

In healthy adult men given calcium and colecalciferol supplementation, no effects were seen on rates of bone mineral loss from either the spine or the radius, despite increased urine calcium excretion and suppressed PTH levels.[97] However, men in this study had a high baseline dietary calcium intake (>1100 mg/day). Calcium supplementation in a calcium-deficient population might prove to be more effective, as has been shown in women.[98]

In a recent study of calcium and colecalciferol supplementation to elderly men with calcium 500mg and colecalciferol 700 IU daily for 3 years,[42] spinal and femoral neck BMD increased by ≈1% in the first year of treatment only. In contrast, differences of 1% in total body BMC compared with age-matched men occurred in the second to third study years. Non-vertebral fractures were less common in calcium-colecalciferol treatment group in women, but not in men.

Two studies have examined the effects of testosterone replacement in healthy elderly men. One study showed that parenteral testosterone supplementation reduced urinary hydroxyproline excretion and increased spinal BMD.[56] A larger study of transdermal testosterone, however, did not reveal any changes in more up-to-date biochemical bone markers.[57]

Rudman et al.[94] found that in addition to beneficial effects of lean mass, fat mass and skin thickness, vertebral BMD was increased significantly by 1.6% over 6 months with growth hormone administration, but there were no changes in radial and proximal femoral density. Thus, GH is a potential, but unproven, agent in the treatment of osteoporosis; unfortunately, its use is associated with adverse effects and considerable expense.

7. Conclusions

No effective treatment to reduce fracture rates has yet been established for men with osteoporosis. While secondary causes of osteoporosis in men should first be excluded and appropriately treated, there is a need for a treatment to increase bone density and decrease fracture rates where no such cause can be identified in men.

There have been three double-blind, placebo-controlled trials of osteoporosis therapies in men. Intermittent low-dose sodium monophosphate and calcium reduced vertebral fractures in men with idiopathic osteoporosis. Dietary calcium supplementation in elderly men results in small, but significant increases in bone density at most sites. However, it is likely that both non-sex hormonal antiresorptive drugs (calcitonin, bisphosphonates and calcitriol) and bone formation-stimulating drugs (e.g. PTH) that are efficacious in women will also be effective in men. This is largely because the pathophysiological mechanisms of osteoporosis and the mechanisms of action of these drugs on bone and mineral metabolism are similar in men and women.

Randomised, double-blind, placebo-controlled trials are currently being conducted comparing alendronic acid with calcium; IGF-1 with placebo; PTH with calcium; and calcitriol with calcium in men with idiopathic osteoporosis. These 6-month to 3-year studies will determine whether any of these drugs are effective in increasing lumbar spine, femoral neck and total body bone density in men, as well as examining their effects on bone turnover markers. It is uncertain whether they will have adequate power to detect differnces in fracture rates.

Osteoporosis in men will become an increasing worldwide public health problem over the next 20 years and for this reason it is vital that safe and efficacious therapies become available to treat men with this disabling condition. Most importantly, effective public health measures also need to be established and targeted to those men at risk of developing the disease.

Acknowledgements

I would like to thank Associate Professor Jeffrey Zajac for his critical appraisal of the manuscript.

References

1. Orwoll ES, Klein RF. Osteoporosis in men. Endocr Rev 1995; 16: 87-116
2. Cooper C, Campion G, Melton LJ. Hip fractures in the elderly: a worldwide projection. Osteoporosis Int 1992; 2: 285-9
3. Cooper C, Atkinson EJ, O'Fallon MW, et al. Incidence of clinically diagnosed vertebral fractures: a population-based study in Rochester, Minnesota 1985-1989. J Bone Miner Res 1992; 7: 221-7
4. Seeman E. Osteoporosis in men: epidemiology, pathophysiology and treatment possibilities. Am J Med 1993; 95: 225-85
5. Parfitt AM, Duncan H. Metabolic bone disease affecting the spine. In: Rothman R, editor. The spine. 2nd ed. Philadelphia: Saunders, 1982; 775-905
6. Jones G, Nguyen T, Sambrook PN, et al. Symptomatic fracture incidence in elderly men and women: the Dubbo Osteoporosis Epidemiology Study (DOES). Osteoporosis Int 1994; 4: 277-82
7. Melton LJ III, Thamer M, Ray NF, et al. Fractures attributable to osteoporosis: report from the National Osteoporosis Foundation. J Bone Miner Res 1997; 12: 16-23
8. Poor G, Atkinson EJ, Lewallen DG, et al. Age-related hip fractures in men: clinical spectrum and short term outcomes. Osteoporosis Int 1995; 5: 419-26
9. Burger H, Van Daele PLA, Grasluis K, et al. Vertebral deformities and functional impairment in men and women. J Bone Miner Res 1997; 12: 152-7
10. Randell A, Sambrook PN, Nguyen TV, et al. Direct clinical and welfare costs of osteoporotic fractures in elderly men and women. Osteoporosis Int 1995; 5: 427-32
11. Ross PD, Kim S, Wasnich RD. Bone density predicts vertebral fracture risk in both men and women [abstract]. J Bone Miner Res 1996; 11 (S1): A132
12. Nguyen TV, Eisman JA, Kelly PJ, et al. Risk factors for osteoporotic fractures in elderly men. Am J Epidemiol 1996; 144: 255-63
13. Poor G, Atkinson EJ, O'Fallon WM, et al. Predictors of hip fractures in elderly men. J Bone Miner Res 1995; 10: 1900-7
14. Stanley HL, Schmitt BP, Poses RM, et al. Does hypogonadism contribute to the occurrence of a minimal trauma hip fracture. J Am Geriatr Soc 1991; 39: 766-71
15. Cooper C, Coupland C, Mitchell M. Rheumatoid arthritis corticosteroid therapy and hip fracture. Ann Rheum Dis 1995; 54: 49-52

16. Christian JC, Yu P-L, Slemenda CW, et al. Hereditability of bone mass: a longitudinal study of aging male twins. Am J Hum Genet 1989; 44: 429-33
17. Pocock NA, Eisman JA, Hopper JL, et al. Genetic determinants of bone mass in adults. J Clin Invest 1987; 80: 706-10
18. Snow-Harter CR, Whalen K, Mybrugh S, et al. Bone mineral density, muscle strength, and recreational exercise in men. J Bone Miner Res 1992; 7: 1291-6
19. Slemenda CW, Christian JC, Reed T, et al. Long-term bone loss in men: effects of genetic and environmental factors. Ann Intern Med 1992; 117: 286-91
20. Jones G, Nguyen T, Sambrook P, et al. Progressive loss of bone in the femoral neck in elderly people: longitudinal findings from the Dubbo Osteoporosis Epidemiology Study. BMJ 1995; 309: 691-5
21. Riggs BL, Melton LJ III. Involutional osteoporosis. N Engl J Med 1986; 314: 1676-86
22. Garn SM, Sullivan TV, Decker SA, et al. Continuing bone expansion and increasing bone loss over a two-decade period in men and women from a total community sample. Am J Hum Biol 1992; 4: 57-67
23. Mosekilde L, Mosekilde L. Normal vertebral body size and compressive strength relations to age and to vertebral and iliac bone compressive strength. Bone 1986; 7: 207-12
24. Compston JE, Mellish RWE, Groucher P, et al. Structural mechanisms of trabecular bone loss in men. Bone Miner 1989; 6: 339-50
25. Beck TJ, Ruff CB, Scott Jr WW, et al. Sex differences in geometry of femoral neck with aging: a structural analysis of bone mineral data. Calcif Tissue Int 1992; 50: 24-9
26. Ebeling PR, Petrson JM, Riggs BL. Utility of type I procollagen propeptide assays for assessing abnormalities in metabolic bone diseases. J Bone Miner Res 1992; 7: 1243-50
27. Tsai KS, Pan WH, Hsu SH, et al. Sexual differences in bone markers and bone mineral density of normal Chinese. Calcif Tissue Int 1996; 59: 454-60
28. Schneider DL, Barett-Connor EL. Urinary N-telopeptide levels discriminate normal osteopenic and osteoporotic bone mineral density. Arch Intern Med 1997; 157: 1241-5
29. Sone T, Miyake M, Takeda N, et al. Urinary excretion of type I N-telopeptides in healthy Japanese adults: age-and sex-related changes and reference limits. Bone 1995; 17: 335-9
30. Krall EA, Dawson-Hughes B, Hirst K, et al. Bone mineral density and biochemical markers of bone turnover in healthy elderly men and women. J Gerontol A Biol Sci Med Sci 1997; 52: M61-7
31. Endres DB, Morgan CH, Garry PJ, et al. Age-related changes in serum immunoreactive parathyroid hormone and its biological action in healthy men and women. J Clin Endocrinol Metab 1987; 65: 724-31
32. Orwoll ES, Meier DE. Alterations in calcium, vitamin D, and parathyroid hormone physiology in normal men with aging: relationship to the development of senile osteopenia. J Clin Endocrinol Metab 1986; 63: 1262-9
33. Slovik DM, Adams JS, Neer RM, et al. Deficient production of 1,25-dihydroxy vitamin D in elderly osteoporotic patients. N Engl J Med 1981; 305: 372-4
34. Halloran BP, Portale AA, Lonergan ET, et al. Production and metabolic clearance of 1,25-dihydroxy vitamin D in men: effect of advancing age. J Clin Endocrinol Metab 1990; 70: 318-23
35. Ebeling PR, Sandgren ME, Di Magno EP, et al. Evidence of an age-related decrease in intestinal responsiveness to vitamin D: relationship between serum 1,25-dihydroxyvitamin D_3 and intestinal vitamin D receptors in normal women. J Clin Endocrinol Metab 1992; 75: 176-82
36. Kinyamu HK, Gallagher JC, Prahl JM, et al. Association between intestinal vitamin D receptor, calcium absorption, and serum 1,25 dihydroxyvitamin D in normal young and elderly women. J Bone Miner Res 1997; 12: 922-8
36a. Need AG, Morris HA, Horowitz M, et al. Intestinal calcium absorption in men with spinal osteoporosis. Clin Endocrinol 1998; 48: 163-8
37. Morrison NA, Qi JC, Tokita A, Kelly PJ, et al. Prediction of bone density from vitamin D receptor alleles. Nature 1994; 367: 284-7
38. Krall EA, Parry P, Lichter JB, et al. Vitamin D receptor alleles and rates of bone loss: influences of years since menopause and calcium intake. J Bone Miner Res 1995; 10: 978-84
39. Kroger H, Laitinen K. Bone mineral density measured by dual-energy x-ray absorptiometry in normal men. Eur J Clin Invest 1992; 22: 454-60
40. Kelly PJ, Pocock NA, Sambrook PN, et al. Dietary calcium, sex hormones and bone mineral density in men. BMJ 1990; 300: 1361-4
41. Looker AC, Harris TB, Madans JH, et al. Dietary calcium and hip fracture risk: the NHANES epidemiologic follow-up study. Osteoporosis Int 1993; 3: 177-84
42. Dawson-Hughes B, Harris SS, Krall EA, et al. Effect of calcium and vitamin D supplementation on bone density in men and women 65 years of age or older. N Engl J Med 1997; 337: 670-6
42a. Ducy P, Amling M, Takeda S, et al. Leptin inhibits bone formation through a hypothalamic relay: a central control of bone mass. Cell 2000; 100: 197-207
43. Francis RM, Peacock M, Marshall DH, et al. Spinal osteoporosis in men. Bone Miner 1989; 5: 347-57
44. MacAdams MR, White RH, Chipps BE. Reduction of serum testosterone levels during chronic glucocorticoid therapy. Ann Intern Med 1986; 104: 648-51
45. Chavassieux P, Serre CM, Vernaud P. *In vitro* evaluation of dose-effect of ethanol on human osteoblastic cells. Bone Miner 1993; 22: 95-103
46. Diamond T, Stiel D, Lunzer M, et al. Ethanol reduced bone formation and may cause osteoporosis. Am J Med 1989; 86: 282-8
47. Hopper JL, Seeman E. The bone density of female twins discordant for smoking. N Engl J Med 1994; 330: 387-92
48. Seeman E, Melton LJ III. Risk factors for spinal osteoporosis in males. Am J Med 1983; 75: 977-83
49. Francis RM, Peacock M, Marshall DH, et al. Spinal osteoporosis in men. Bone Miner 1989; 5: 347-57
50. Francis RM, Peacock M. Osteoporosis in hypogonadal men: role of decreased plasma 1,25-dihydroxy vitamin D, calcium malabsorption and low bone formation. Bone 1986; 261-8

51. Parfitt AM, Duncan H. Metabolic bone disease affecting the spine. In: Rothman R, editor. The spine. 2nd ed. Philadelphia: Saunders, 1982: 775-905
52. Nordin BEC, Aaron J, Speed R, et al. Bone formation and resorption as the determinants of trabecular bone volume in normal and osteoporotic men. Scott Med J 1984; 29: 171-5
53. Aaron JE, Francis RM, Peacock M, et al. Contrasting microanatomy of idiopathic and corticosteroid-induced osteoporosis. Clin Orthop 1989; 243: 294-305
54. Ferrini RL, Barrett-Connort E. Sex hormones and age: a cross-sectional study of testosterone and estradiol and their bioavailable fractions in community-dwelling men. Am J Epidemiol 1998; 15: 750-4
55. Clarke BL, Ebeling PR, Wahner HW, et al. Steroid hormones influence bone histomorphometric parameters in healthy men [abstract]. Calcif Tissue Int 1994; 54: 334
56. Tenover JS. Effects of testosterone supplementation in the aging male. J Clin Endocrinol Metab 1992; 75: 1092-8
57. Orwoll ES, Oviatt S. Transdermal testosterone supplementation in normal older men [abstract]. Proc Endocr Soc 1992; A1071
58. Jackson JA, Kleerekoper M. Bone histomorphometry in hypogonadal and eugonadal men with spinal osteoporosis. J Clin Endocrinol Metab 1987; 65: 53-8
59. Stepan JJ, Lachman M. Castrated men with bone loss: effect of calcitonin on biochemical indices of bone remodelling. J Clin Endocrinol Metab 1989; 69: 523-7
60. Katznelson L, Finklestein JS, Schoenfeld DA, et al. Increase in bone density and lean body mass during testosterone administration in men with acquired hypogonadism. J Clin Endocrinol Metab 1996; 81: 4358-65
61. Devogelaer JP, De Cooman S, Nagant de Deuxchaisnes C. Low bone mass in hypogonadal males: effect of testosterone substitution therapy, a densitometric study. Maturitas 1992; 15: 17-23
62. Bagchi MK, Tsai MJ, O'Malley BW, et al. Analysis of the mechanism of steroid hormone receptor-dependent gene activation in cell-free systems. Endocr Rev 1992; 13: 525-35
63. Lubahn DB, Joseph DR, Sar M, et al. The human androgen receptor: complementary deoxyribonucleic acid cloning, sequence analysis, and gene expression in prostate. Mol Endocrinol 1988; 2: 1265-75
64. Edwards A, Hammond HA, Jin L, et al. Genetic variation at five trimeric and tetrameric tandem repeat loci in four human population groups. Genomics 1992; 12: 241-53
65. Sleddens HF, Oostra BA, Brinkmann AO, et al. Trinucleotide (GGN) repeat polymorphism in the human androgen receptor (AR) gene. Hum Mol Genet 1995; 2: 493-7
66. Kazemi-Esfarjani P, Trifiro M, Pinsky L. Evidence for a repressive function of the long polyglutamine tract in the human androgen receptor: possible pathogenic relevance for the (CAG)n-expanded neuropathies. Hum Mol Genet 1995; 4: 523-7
67. Cohen P, Peehl DM, Graves HC, et al. Biological effects of prostate specific antigens as an insulin-like growth factor binding protein-3 protease. J Endocrinol 1994; 142: 407-15
68. Brass AL, Barnard J, Patai BL, et al. Androgen up-regulates epidermal growth factor receptor expression and binding affinity in PC3 cell lines expressing human androgen receptor. Cancer Res 1995; 54: 3197-203
69. Wilding G, Valverius E, Knabbe C, et al. Role of transforming growth factor in a human prostate cancer cell growth. Prostate 1989; 15: 1-12
70. Marcelli M, Haidacher SJ, Plymate SR, et al. Altered growth and insulin-like growth factor binding protein-3 production in PC3 prostate carcinoma cells stably transfected with a constitutively active androgen receptor complementary deoxyribonucleic acid. Endocrinology 1995; 136: 1040-8
71. Ebeling PR, Jones JD, O'Fallon WM, et al. Short-term effects of recombinant hIGF-I on bone turnover in normal women. J Clin Endocrinol Metab 1993; 77: 1384-7
72. Kurland ES, Rosen CJ, Cosman F, et al. Insulin-like growth factor-I in men with idiopathic osteoporosis. J Clin Endocrinol Metab 1997; 82: 2799-805
73. Spotila LD, Constantinos CD, Sereda L, et al. Mutation in a gene for type I procollagen (COL1A2) in a woman with postmenopausal osteoporosis: evidence for phenotypic and genetic overlap with mild osteogenesis imperfecta. Proc Natl Acad Sci U S A 1991; 88: 5423-7
74. Grant SFA, Reid DM, Ralston SH. Osteoporotic fracture and reduced bone density related to a polymorphism in the transcriptional control region of the collagen type I a 1 gene [abstract]. J Bone Miner Res 1995; 10 (S1): A106
75. Vanderscheueren D, Van Herck E, De Coster R, et al. Aromatisation of androgens is important for skeletal maintenance of aged male rats. Calcif Tissue Int 1996; 59: 179-83
76. Smith EP, Boyd J, Frank GR, et al. Estrogen resistance caused by a mutation in the estrogen-receptor gene in a man. N Engl J Med 1994; 331: 1056-61
77. Ke-nan Q, Fisher CR, Grumbach MM, et al. Aromatase deficiency in a male subject: characterization of a mutation in the CYP gene in an affected family [abstract]. Endocrinol Soc 1995; A P3-27
78. Bilezikian JP, Morishima A, Bell J, et al. Increased bone mass as a result of estrogen therapy in a man with aromatase deficiency. N Engl J Med 1998; 339: 599-603
79. Slemenda CW, Longcope C, Zhou L, et al. Sex steroids and bone mass in older men: positive associations with serum estrogens and negative associations with androgens. J Clin Invest 1997; 100: 1755-9
80. Van Kesteren, Lips P, Deville W, et al. The effect of one-year cross-sex hormonal treatment on bone metabolism and serum insulin-like growth factor-I treatment in transsexuals. J Clin Endocrinol Metab 1996; 81: 2227-32
81. Lubahn DB, Moyer JS, Golding TS, et al. Alteration of reproductive function but not prenatal sexual development after insertional disruption of the mouse estrogen receptor gene. Proc Natl Acad Sci U S A 1993; 90: 11162-6
82. Kobayashi S, Inoue S, Hosoi T, et al. Association of bone mineral density with polymorphism of the estrogen receptor gene. J Bone Miner Res 1996; 11: 306-11
82a. Ringe JD, Dorst A, Kipshoven C, et al. Avoidance of vertebral fractures in men with idiopathic osteoporosis by a three year therapy with calcium and low-dose intermittent monofluorophosphate. Osteoporosis Int 1998; 8: 47-52

83. Agrawal R, Wallack S, Cohn S, et al. Calcitonin treatment of osteoporosis. In: Pecile A, editor. Calcitonin. Amsterdam: Exerpta Medica, 1981; 540: 237
84. Selby PL, Rehman MT, Economou G, et al. Etidronate in male osteoporosis: evidence for a site-specific action [abstract]. In: Christiansen C, editor. Osteoporosis 1993. Aalborg: Aalborg APS, 1993: 197
85. Anderson FH, Francis RM, Bishop JC, et al. Effect of intermittent cyclical disodium etidronate therapy on bone mineral density in men with vertebral fractures. Age Ageing 1997; 26: 359-65
86. Orme SM, Simpson M, Stewart SP, et al. Comparison of changes in idiopathic and secondary osteoporosis following therapy with disodium etidronate and high dose calcium supplementation. Clin Endocrinol (Oxf) 1994; 41: 245-50
87. Anderson FH, Francis RM, Peaston RT, et al. Androgen supplementation in eugonadal men with osteoporosis: effects of six months treatment on markers of bone formation and bone resorption. J Bone Miner Res 1997; 12: 472-8
88. Slovik DM, Rosenthal DI, Doppelt SH, et al. Restoration of spinal bone in osteoporotic men by treatment with human parathyroid hormone (1-34) and 1,25-dihydroxy vitamin D. J Bone Miner Res 1986; 1: 377-81
88a. Ebeling PR, Yeung S, Poon C, et al. Effects of baseline active calcium absorption on bone mineral density (BMD) responses to calcitriol or calcium treatment in men with idiopathic osteoporosis. J Bone Miner Res 1999; 14 Suppl 1: A 414
89. Reeve J, Davis UM, Hesp R, et al. Human parathyroid peptide treatment of osteoporosis substantially increases spinal trabecular bone (with observations on the effects of sodium fluoride therapy). BMJ 1990; 301: 314-8, 477
90. Lindsay R, Cosman F, Shen V, et al. Bone mass increments induced by PTH treatment can be maintained by oestrogen [abstract]. J Bone Miner Res 1995; 10 (S2): A200
91. Hodsman AB, Steer BM, Fraher L, et al. Bone densitometric and histomorphometric responses to sequential human parathyroid hormone (1-38) and salmon calcitonin in osteoporotic patients. Bone Miner 1991; 14: 67-83
91a. Orwoll E, Ettinger M, Weiss S, et al. Alendronate treatment of osteoporosis in men. J Bone Miner Res 1999; 14 Suppl 1: A1205
92. Greenspan SL, Holland S, Maitland-Ramsey L, et al. Nocturnal stimulation of parathyroid hormone: a mechanism to explain the continued improvement in bone mineral density following alendronate therapy [abstract]. J Bone Miner Res 1995; 10 (S1): A449
93. Finkelsten JS, Klibanski A, Schafer EH, et al. Parathyroid hormone for the prevention of bone loss induced by oestrogen deficiency. N Engl J Med 1994; 331: 1618-23
94. Rudman D, Feller AG, Hoskote S, et al. Effects of human growth hormone in men over 60 years old. N Engl J Med 1990; 323: 1-6
95. Holloway L, Kohlmeier L, Kent K, et al. Skeletal effects of cyclic recombinant human growth hormone and salmon calcitonin in osteopenic postmenopausal women. J Clin Endocrinol Metab 1997; 82: 1111-7
96. Ghiron LJ, Thompson JL, Holloway L, et al. Effects of recombinant insulin-like growth factor-1 and growth hormone on bone turnover in elderly women. J Bone Miner Res 1995; 10: 1844-52
97. Orwoll ES, Oviatt SK, McClung MR, et al. The rate of bone mineral loss in normal men and the effects of calcium and cholecalciferol supplementation. Ann Intern Med 1990; 112: 29-34
98. Dawson-Hughes B, Dallal GE, Krall EA, et al. A controlled trial of the effect of calcium supplementation on bone density in postmenopausal women. N Engl J Med 1990; 323: 878-83

Correspondence: Dr *P.R. Ebeling*, Department of Diabetes and Endocrinology, Royal Melbourne Hospital, Victoria 3050, Australia.
E-mail: p.ebeling@medicine.unimelb.edu.au

Pathogenesis and Treatment of Glucocorticoid-Induced Osteoporosis

Paula J. Rackoff[1] and *Clifford J. Rosen*[2]

1 Department of Rheumatology, Beth Israel Hospital, New York, New York, USA
2 Department of Medicine, St Joseph Hospital, Bangor, Maine, USA

Glucocorticoid-induced osteoporosis was first described more than half a century ago.[1] However, the extent of this problem is more evident today because awareness of osteoporosis has increased and bone densitometry has become more accessible. Indeed, of all the secondary causes of low bone mass, glucocorticoid-induced osteoporosis remains the most common but the most frustrating to manage.[2] Advances in our understanding of the bone remodelling unit have helped us to appreciate the severity of the skeletal bone loss induced by glucocorticoids.

Moreover, as the pathogenesis of several rheumatic disorders has become clearer, the effects of these diseases on bone have also been elucidated. Unfortunately, older individuals, who often have a very low bone mineral density (BMD), are more susceptible to rheumatic disorders and are more likely to receive glucocorticoids. Thus, the combination of aging and glucocorticoid use, against a background of an underlying disorder such as rheumatoid arthritis (RA), establishes a vicious cycle of rapid bone loss, fracture, pain, disability and loss of function. In this article, we examine the mechanisms associated with bone loss due to aging and glucocorticoid use, the epidemiology of corticosteroid use among the elderly and the potential treatment regimens.

1. Pathogenesis of Aging-Related Osteoporosis

The incidence of osteoporotic fractures rises exponentially with age.[3] In part, this has been related to a higher rate of falling among individuals aged >70 years. However, age, independent of the number of falls, remains a potent risk factor for osteoporosis.[4] This can be traced to two inter-related determinants: (i) an age-associated decline in BMD; and (ii) a marked reduction in the structural integrity of the skeleton.[5,6] The pathogenetic factors that account for these changes (e.g. bodyweight loss, undernutrition, hypogonadism, calcium deficiency, genetics and others) have often been described. For example, it is known that after the age of 50 years, in both men and women, BMD declines at a rate of 0.5 to 1% per year.[7] In women, the rates of bone loss may be higher during the immediate postmenopausal period.[8] Also, bone loss may actually accelerate after the age of 70 years, even in eugonadal individuals.[9] In fact, biochemical markers of bone turnover in women aged >70 years are twice as high as those noted in the fifth, sixth and seventh decades.[9,10] It is likely, although not proven, that increased bone resorption contributes to both a decline in bone mass and a decrease in the structural integrity of bone.[10]

There are several mechanisms involved in aging-related bone loss and, not surprisingly, each one is also present in patients receiving glucocorticoids. At the level of the bone remodelling unit, bone resorption is accelerated while bone formation is impaired.[11] This produces a marked uncoupling in the remodelling cycle and results in a net deficit of new bone. Calcium deficiency increases bone resorption and may be the most common cause of rapidly accelerated bone loss in the elderly.[12] The dietary intake of calcium in older individuals is often 1 g/day lower than the recommended amount.[13] This alone can produce secondary hyperparathyroidism, which, in turn, stimulates bone resorption.

In elderly individuals, vitamin D deficiency often coexists with a low calcium intake.[14] This is especially true for nursing home residents, in whom exposure to sunlight is minimal. The combination of low vitamin D and reduced calcium intakes markedly exacerbates bone loss, leading to a higher overall fracture risk. Poor nutrition, immobility and muscle atrophy can also contribute to a higher rate of bone resorption as elderly and frail individuals become more infirm and exert less force on their skeleton.[15]

In addition to the alterations in bone resorption, bone formation is also affected by aging.[16] Bone forming cells (osteoblasts) from older individuals have a reduced proliferative capacity, and they are less capable of forming new bone *in vitro*.[17] The mechanisms responsible for these changes are not clear. Nevertheless, it is known that levels of insulin-like growth factor–I (IGF-I), a potent mitogenic and differentiative factor, decline with age in the skeleton and in the serum.[18] Changes in serum levels of IGF-I may be attributable to reduced growth hormone secretion, although undernutrition is also a factor.[19]

Moreover, levels of the inhibitory IGF binding protein (IGFBP)-4 rise dramatically in advanced age and in catabolic states.[20] Serum IGFBP-4 levels are also very high in patients with secondary hyperparathyroidism.[21] The level of IGFBP-5, an IGF binding protein that enhances IGF-I activity, declines with increasing age.[22] Thus, reduced bone formation, a characteristic of the aging remodelling unit, could result from dramatically lower levels of IGF-I and IGFBP-5 and higher levels of IGFBP-4. In individuals who are deficient in calcium and vitamin D, decreased bone formation and increased bone resorption may result in bone loss from the trabecular skeleton of 3 to 5% per year.

In summary, any process that uncouples the bone remodelling system results in a rapid decline in BMD. Moreover, skeletal integrity can be further compromised by accelerated bone resorption. These processes, combined with alterations in the IGF regulatory system, are likely to be responsible for the pathogenesis of age-related fractures. As noted in sections 2.1 and 2.2, glucocorticoid use causes similar changes at all levels, and their use in long term treatment results in tremendously increased skeletal fragility (table I).

Table I. Mechanisms of osteoporotic bone loss in the elderly and in patients receiving glucocorticoids

Elderly	Glucocorticoid recipients
↓ Bone formation	↓ Bone formation
↑ Bone resorption	↑ Bone resorption
↓ Skeletal mass	↓ Skeletal mass
Poor nutrition	Catabolic state
↓ Calcium intake	
Vitamin D deficiency	Impaired vitamin D metabolism
Micronutrient deficiencies	? Micronutrient deficiencies
Hypogonadism	Primary or secondary hypogonadism
↑ Parathyroid hormone	↑ Parathyroid hormone

↑ = increased; ↓ = reduced; ? = possible.

2. Pathogenesis of Glucocorticoid-Induced Bone Loss

Aging-associated bone loss provides an example of a modest uncoupling in the bone remodelling unit that occurs as a result of changes in both bone resorption and formation. Glucocorticoid-induced osteoporosis is the extreme example of a syndrome that is characterised by a major imbalance in the remodelling process, leading to greater bone fragility.[23] As noted in table I, glucocorticoids have profound effects on the skeleton that resemble those seen with aging, although the former are of much greater magnitude. The effects of corticosteroids on bone are best considered as either direct or indirect.

2.1 Direct Effects

Glucocorticoids inhibit a diverse range of bone cell functions, including cell growth, multiplication and differentiation, alkaline phosphatase activity, type I collagen production and the synthesis of noncollagen proteins.[24] In particular, supraphysiological dosages of corticosteroids have a profound effect on osteoblasts. This results in the consistent histomorphometric finding in patients receiving glucocorticoids of a decreased mean wall thickness, as less bone is formed during each remodelling cycle.[25] Collagen synthesis is also dramatically affected by high dosages of glucocorticoids through a direct inhibition of collagen type Iα mRNA in osteoblasts.[26]

High dosages of glucocorticoids also inhibit IGF-I mRNA expression in rat tibiae, in organ cultures of fetal calvariae and in human osteoblasts.[27] These changes are accompanied by a down-regulation of IGFBP-5 (a stimulatory IGFBP) and an up-regulation of IGFBP-1 (another inhibitory IGF binding protein) and IGFBP-4.[28] Glucocorticoids also inhibit the expression of many noncollagenous skeletal proteins, the most prominent of which is osteocalcin.[29] Recent preliminary studies suggest that high dosages of corticosteroids stimulate apoptosis in bone forming cells. All of these changes lead to a profound reduction in bone formation within weeks of the initiation of glucocorticoid therapy. Such changes are evident from biochemical markers of bone turnover, BMD measurements and histomorphometry.

2.2 Indirect Effects

Unfortunately, the effects of glucocorticoids on bone formation are not the only sequelae of this class of drugs. There are multiple *in vivo* actions of glucocorticoids that contribute to rapid bone loss, especially within the first year of treatment. For example, corticosteroids can impair the 1α-hydroxylation of 25-hydroxycholecalciferol (25-hydroxyvitamin D_3; calcifediol) in some clinical situations, leading to a state of relative vitamin D deficiency.[30] This, in turn, can result in secondary hyperparathyroidism, leading to an increase in bone resorption. Similarly, glucocorticoids can block calcium absorption in the gut and increase urinary calcium excretion, both of which aggravate secondary hyperparathyroidism.[31]

Moreover, corticosteroids can affect skeletal prostaglandins and certain cytokines, further driving osteoclast-mediated bone resorption, and thereby increasing the magnitude of bone loss.[32] High dosages of corticosteroids also impair muscle function, which results in disuse atrophy, another factor that indirectly increases bone resorption and decreases bone formation.[33] Finally, primary and secondary hypogonadism are common in patients receiving high dosages of glucocorticoids for a prolonged period.[34] Similar to during the menopause, hormonal deprivation in both men and women receiving glucocorticoids results in increased cytokine release and accelerated bone resorption.[35]

Thus, glucocorticoid therapy has a profound effect on bone remodelling through both direct and indirect mechanisms. This results in rapid bone loss, especially during the early stages of therapy when high dosages of corticosteroids are employed. To make matters worse, glucocorticoids are often prescribed to older individuals who are already deficient in calcium and vitamin D and in whom, superimposed on this, age-associated processes are occurring in the skeleton. The combination of high dosages of glucocorticoids and an underlying disorder that might have independent deleterious effects on the skeleton makes for a potentially disastrous situation in elderly, frail individuals who are already at risk for fractures.

3. Glucocorticoid Use in Chronic Diseases of the Elderly

Glucocorticoids are extensively used by elderly patients for the treatment of acute and chronic forms of asthma, chronic lung disease, RA and other connective tissue diseases, inflammatory bowel disease and degenerative, inflammatory neurological diseases. Intervention with glucocorticoids often decreases both the morbidity and mortality from these diseases; however, the adverse effects of glucocorticoids, such as osteoporosis, carry their own risk for morbidity and mortality. In the geriatric population, this additional cause of osteoporosis can have devastating consequences.

The clinical significance of osteoporosis lies in the fractures that ensue. Fractures of the spine and forearm are associated with increased morbidity, but it is hip fracture that has a high rate of mortality (15 to 20%), particularly in elderly men and women.[36] Older age, male gender and poorer general health are associated with an increased in-hospital mortality.[37] In fact, among those with a hip fracture attributable to glucocorticoid use, mortality rates for men aged >50 years range from 5 to 9%, compared with 1 to 3% for age-matched women.[38] Over a lifetime, the BMD of the femoral neck decreases by 58 and 39% in women and men, respectively, independent of corticosteroid use.[10,39] By the time a White woman reaches menopause, her remaining lifetime risk of hip fracture reaches 17%.[3,6] Add to that a nearly equal risk of vertebral, forearm and other fractures, and the combined risk is 30 to 40%.[40] Moreover, it is certain that these numbers will increase in the next 50 years. Globally, there are now an estimated 323 million people over the age of 65 years, and this number is expected to increase to 1555 million by the year 2050.[41]

The general consensus is that moderate-to-high dosage glucocorticoid therapy is associated with increased bone turnover and an increased risk of fracture. It is not known whether there is a threshold dosage for corticosteroids below which osteopenia does not develop. Most studies, however, support the view that dosages of prednisone ≥7.5 mg/day result in an increased fracture risk.[42-46] Furthermore, alternate-day glucocorticoid regimens have not been shown to reduce the risk of osteoporosis, and high dosages of inhaled corticosteroids can also cause bone loss.[45-47] Overall, it is the cumulative dose of corticosteroids that correlates with bone loss. Hence, up to 40% of patients receiving long term glucocorticoid treatment develop fractures.[42-46]

Despite the risk of fracture associated with corticosteroids, most people, and particularly the elderly, do not receive treatment for bone loss and are unable to access preventive therapy. Walsh et al.[48] conducted a community survey of 65 000 inhabitants of Nottinghamshire, England. In this population, 0.5% (303 patients) had been receiving oral corticosteroids for at least 3 months (mean duration of treatment 3 years) at a mean dosage equivalent to prednisone 8 mg/day. Surprisingly, only 14% of the 303 patients had received medication to prevent osteoporosis over the course of the 4-year study.[48]

Corticosteroids are often the mainstay of treatment in chronic rheumatological conditions. The incidence of RA in the adult population is approximately 1%; its prevalence increases with advancing age up to the seventh decade.[49,50] Giant cell arteritis and polymyalgia rheumatica are essentially limited to individuals aged >50 years, and the incidence of these conditions increases with age.[51] One of the criteria for the diagnosis of RA is juxta-articular bone loss, which is seen early on in the course of RA. It is believed that cytokines (interleukin-1, tumour necrosis factor and interferon-γ) released from activated lymphocytes and macrophages are major mediators of localised osteoporosis. Generalised osteoporosis is also seen in RA, and involves both cortical and trabecular bone. The aetiology of this diffuse osteoporosis is multifactorial and includes: (i) decreased physical activity and increased immobility; (ii) poor nutritional status; (iii) impaired absorption of calcium; (iv) postmenopausal status in women; and (v) medications, most notably corticosteroids.

Patients with RA carry a 2-fold increased risk of osteoporosis, both at the spine and hip, that cannot be explained by the use of corticosteroids or by disease activity.[52,53] Although both trabecular and skeletal bone are affected by corticosteroids, patients with active inflammatory disease were shown by Laan et al.[54] to have increased vertebral (trabecular) bone loss; patients with more functional impairment, particularly those with poor mobility, had a greater risk of femoral bone loss. Cooper et al.[44] observed that patients with RA who were receiving corticosteroids had a 5-fold increase in the number of vertebral deformities compared with those not receiving glucocorticoids. Dykman et al.[55] reported a 50% increase in the incidence of fractures in patients with RA who were receiving prednisone, compared with RA patients in the same study not receiving prednisone, most being vertebral fractures.

Bone loss caused by glucocorticoid therapy appears to be most rapid during the first 6 to 12 months of therapy, in both men and women. Hall et al.[56] assessed BMD in postmenopausal women with RA and the relative influences of disease activity, disability, and past and current use of corticosteroids. Thirty-five of 195 postmenopausal women with RA who had discontinued corticosteroid treatment had a BMD at all sites which was similar to that in patients who had never used corticosteroids. Although the cumulative dose among previous users was similar to that among current low-dose users, the former group had a greater BMD (absolute percentage differences 6.4 and 5% at the lumbar spine and femur, respectively) than the latter. This supports the view that recovery from corticosteroid-induced osteoporosis is possible with cessation of treatment.[56]

The magnitude of corticosteroid-induced osteoporosis in RA can surely be extrapolated to other connective tissue disorders and other diseases that necessitate long term corticosteroid treatment. Juxta-articular osteoporosis, however, is much more common in RA. Undoubtedly, the inflammatory components of RA (i.e. cytokines and various growth factors) can induce localised bone loss. However, it remains to be established whether activation of the immune system, and of various cytokines systemically, can cause generalised osteoporosis in patients with RA or other connective tissue disorders.

4. Therapeutic Interventions for Glucocorticoid-Induced Osteoporosis in the Elderly

The best treatment for osteoporosis is to prevent bone loss before the disease has become established. Several longitudinal studies of patients with Cushing's disease (the result of a corticotrophin–secreting pituitary tumour) have demonstrated that bone loss attributable to longstanding glucocorticoid excess can be reversed after surgical cure.[57] Observational, anecdotal and randomised studies in patients receiving low to high dosages of glucocorticoids confirm that bone loss can be arrested once the corticosteroids have been discontinued.[44,55,56,58]

Table II. Therapeutic options for glucocorticoid-induced osteoporosis

Agent	Mechanism
Established	
Calcium 1500 mg/day	Improves calcium balance, ↓ resorption
Vitamin D >400 IU/day	Enhances calcium absorption
Thiazide diuretics	↓ Hypercalciuria
Hormone replacement therapy (or androgens)	↓ Resorption
Bisphosphonates[a]	↓ Resorption
Calcitonin	↓ Resorption
Experimental	
Sodium fluoride	Stimulates formation
Growth hormone	Stimulates formation
Parathyroid hormone (intermittent)	Stimulates formation

a The bisphosphonate etidronic acid (etidronate) has been shown to reduce fractures and prevent bone loss in a randomised trial.[59] Very recently, preliminary data (in abstract form only) suggest that alendronic acid 10 mg/day also reduces bone loss in steroid-induced osteoporosis.[60]

↓ = reduces.

Hence, the first goal in preventing the morbid sequelae of this disorder is to lessen the exposure of the patient to glucocorticoids. Maintenance dosages of prednisone <7.5mg on alternate days or gradual tapering with discontinuation are achievable in many circumstances. Calcium and vitamin D should be the cornerstone of all other therapies aimed at reducing bone loss or stimulating bone formation (see table II). In the elderly, high rates of bone loss often exist even before the initiation of glucocorticoids. Hence, antiresorptive therapy should be considered as prophylaxis early in the course of glucocorticoid therapy, rather than later when the disease is well established. In fact, most bone loss attributable to glucocorticoids occurs within the first 6 months of treatment.[61] Thus, there is a need to consider aggressive therapy earlier rather than later.

Unfortunately, few well-designed, randomised, placebo-controlled trials of interventions for established glucocorticoid-induced osteoporosis have been performed. Treatment options that are supported by observational or short, nonrandomised, controlled studies are listed in table II.[62-68] In 1997, however, Adachi et al.[59] demonstrated, in a 2-year, randomised, placebo-controlled trial, that cyclical therapy with etidronic acid (etidronate) 400 mg/day for 2 weeks every 3 months prevented bone loss from the spine and hip among patients requiring long term therapy with glucocorticoids. It also reduced the incidence of vertebral fractures. These data, and those for alendronic acid (alendronate),[60] suggest that the bisphosphonates may be ideal treatments (since they have few systemic adverse effects) for the prevention of corticosteroid-induced bone loss and fractures.

Anabolic agents that stimulate bone formation (table II) are currently being tested in patients with glucocorticoid-induced osteoporosis. The results of those studies in older individuals, where bone formation is already impaired, are awaited with great anticipation. Until those data are available, the best therapy remains preventive treatment (i.e. minimising exposure to corticosteroids) and the administration of calcium and vitamin D, with consideration of the use of hormone replacement therapy or a bisphosphonate if the dosage and duration of corticosteroid treatment is expected to be longer than a few weeks.

References

1. Cushing H. Basophil adenomas of the pituitary body and their clinical manifestations. Bull Johns Hopkins Hosp 1932; 50: 137-95
2. Adler RA, Rosen CJ. Glucocorticoids and osteoporosis. Endocrinol Metab Clin 1994; 23: 641-54
3. Hui SL, Slemenda CW, Johnston CC. Baseline measurement of bone mass predicts fracture in white women. Ann Intern Med 1989; 11: 355-61
4. Kiel DP. The approach to osteoporosis in the elderly patient. In: Rosen CJ, editor. Osteoporosis: diagnostic and therapeutic principles. Totowa (NJ): Humana Press, 1996: 225-39
5. Hui SL, Wiske PS, Norton JA. A prospective study of change in bone mass with age in postmenopausal women. J Chronic Dis 1982; 35: 715-25
6. Cummings SR, Nevitt MC, Browner WS. Risk factors for hip fractures in white women. N Engl J Med 1995; 332: 767-73
7. Greenspan SL, Maitland LA, Myers ER, et al. Femoral bone loss progress with age: a longitudinal study in women over age 65. J Bone Miner Res 1994; 9: 1959-65
8. Ravn P, Hetland ML, Overgaard K, et al. Premenopausal and postmenopausal changes in BMD of the proximal femur measured by dual energy X-ray absorptiometry. J Bone Miner Res 1994; 9: 1975-80
9. Garnero P, Shih WG, Gineyts E, et al. Comparison of new biochemical markers of bone turnover in late postmenopausal osteoporotic women in response to alendronate. J Clin Endocrinol Metab 1994; 79: 1693-700
10. Jones G, Nguyen T, Sambrook P, et al. Progressive loss of bone in the femoral neck in elderly people: longitudinal findings from the Dubbo osteoporosis epidemiology study. BMJ 1994; 309: 691-5
11. Kessenich CR, Rosen CJ. The pathophysiology of osteoporosis. In: Rosen CJ, editor. Osteoporosis: diagnostic and therapeutic principles. Totowa (NJ): Humana Press, 1996: 47-63
12. Dawson-Hughes B, Dallal GE, Krall EA, et al. A controlled trial of the effect of calcium supplementation on bone density in postmenopausal women. N Engl J Med 1990; 323: 878-83
13. NIH Consensus Conference: optimal calcium intake. JAMA 1995; 272: 1942-8
14. Doppelt SH, Neer RM, Daly M, et al. Vitamin D deficiency and osteomalacia in patients with hip fractures. Orthop Trans 1983; 7: 512-3
15. Sowers MF, Wallace RB, Hollis BW, et al. Parameters related to 25 OHD levels in a population based study of women. Am J Clin Nutr 1986; 43: 621-8
16. Rosen CJ. The role of insulin-like growth factor in senescence: clues for interventional strategies in the elderly. Endocrinologist 1996; 6: 102-8
17. Hayden JM, Mohan S, Baylink DJ. The insulin like growth factor system and the coupling of formation to resorption. Bone 1994; 17: 93S-8S
18. Rosen CJ, Donahue LR, Hunter SJ. IGFs and bone: the osteoporosis connection. Proc Soc Exp Biol Med 1994; 206: 83-103
19. Rudman D. Growth hormone, body composition and aging. J Am Geriatr Soc 1985; 33: 800-7
20. Mohan S, Farley J, Baylink DJ. Age-related changes in IGFBP-4 and IGFBP-5 in human serum and bone: implications for the bone loss of aging. Prog Growth Factor Res 1995; 4: 465-73
21. Rosen CJ, Donahue LR, Hunter SJ, et al. The 24/25 kD IGFBP is increased in elderly women with hip and spine fractures. J Clin Endocrinol Metab 1992; 74: 24-7
22. Rajaram S, Baylink DJ, Mohan S. IGFBPs in serum and other biological fluids: regulation and function. Endocr Rev 1997; 18: 801-32
23. Lukert BP, Kream BE. Clinical and basic aspects of glucocorticoid action in bone. In: Bilezikian JP, Raisz LG, Rodan G, editors. Principles of bone biology. San Diego (CA): Academic Press, 1996: 533-48
24. Canalis E. Effect of glucocorticoids on type I collagen synthesis, alkaline phosphatase activity and DNA content in cultured rat calvariae. Endocrinology 1988; 112: 931-5
25. Dempster D. Bone histomorphometry in glucocorticoid-induced osteoporosis. J Bone Miner Res 1989; 4: 137-41
26. Delaney AM, Gabbitas BY, Canalis E. Cortisol down regulates osteoblast alpha I procollagen mRNA by transcriptional and post transcriptional mechanisms. J Cell Biochem 1995; 57: 488-94
27. McCarthy TL, Centrella M, Canalis E. Cortisol inhibits synthesis of IGF-I in skeletal cells. Endocrinology 1990; 126: 1569-75
28. Conover CA, Bale LK, Clarkson JT. Regulation of IGFBP-5 messenger RNA expression and protein availability in rat osteoblastic like cells. Endocrinology 1993; 132: 2525-30
29. Godshalk MF, Downs RW. Effect of short term glucocorticoids on serum osteocalcin in healthy young men. J Bone Miner Res 1988; 3: 113-5
30. Morris HA, Need AG, O'Loughlin PD, et al. Malabsorption of calcium in corticosteroid induced osteoporosis. Calcif Tissue Int 1990; 46: 305-8
31. Suzuki Y, Ichikawa Y, Saito E, et al. Importance of increased urinary calcium excretion in the development of secondary hyperparathyroidism of patients undergoing glucocorticoid therapy. Metabolism 1983; 32: 151-6
32. Delaney AM, Dong Y, Canalis E. Mechanisms of glucocorticoid action in bone cells. J Cell Biochem 1994; 56: 295-302
33. Libanti CR, Baylink DJ. Prevention and treatment of glucocorticoid-induced osteoporosis. Chest 1992; 102: 1426-35
34. MacAdams MR, White RH, Chipps BE. Reduction of serum testosterone levels during chronic glucocorticoid therapy. Ann Intern Med 1986; 104: 648-51
35. Manolagas SC, Jilka RL. Bone marrow, cytokines and bone remodeling. N Engl J Med 1995; 332: 305-11
36. Keene G, Parker M, Pryor G. Mortality and morbidity after hip fractures. BMJ 1993; 307: 1248-50

37. Myers AH, Robinson EG, Van Natta ML, et al. Hip fractures among the elderly: factors associated with in-hospital mortality. Am J Epidemiol 1991; 134: 1128-37
38. US Congress of Technology Assessment. Hip fracture outcomes in people age 50 and over. Washington, DC: US Government Printing Office, 1994: OTA-BP-H 120
39. Riggs BL, Wahner HW, Seeman E, et al. Changes in BMD of the proximal femur and spine with aging. J Clin Invest 1982; 70: 716-23
40. Kanis JA, Delmas P, Burckhardt P, et al. Guidelines for diagnosis and management of osteoporosis. Osteoporos Int 1997; 7: 390-6
41. Cooper C, Campion G, Melton LJ. Hip fractures in the elderly: a worldwide projection. Osteoporos Int 1992; 2: 285-9
42. Verstraeten A, Dequeker J. Vertebral and peripheral bone mineral content and fracture evidence in postmenopausal patients with rheumatoid arthritis: effects of low dose steroids. Ann Rheum Dis 1986; 45: 852-7
43. Michel BA, Block DA, Fries JF. Predictors of fracture in early rheumatoid arthritis. J Rheumatol 1991; 18: 804-8
44. Cooper C, Coupland C, Mitchell M. Rheumatoid arthritis, corticosteroid therapy, and hip fracture. Ann Rheum Dis 1994; 53: 49-52
45. Saag KJ, Koehnke R, Caldwell JR, et al. Low dose long term corticosteroid therapy in rheumatoid arthritis: an analysis of serious adverse events. Am J Med 1994; 96: 115-23
46. Hanania NA, Chapman KR, Sturtridge WC, et al. Dose related decrease in bone density among asthmatic patients treated with inhaled corticosteroids. J Allergy Clin Immunol 1995; 96 (5 Pt 1): 571-9
47. Adinoff AD, Hollister JR. Steroid induced fractures and bone loss in patients with asthma. N Engl J Med 1983; 309: 265-8
48. Walsh LJ, Wong CA, Pringle M, et al. Use of oral glucocorticoids in the community and the prevention of secondary osteoporosis. BMJ 1996; 313: 344-6
49. Lems WF, Jahangier ZN, Jacobs JWG, et al. Vertebral fractures with rheumatoid arthritis patients treated with corticosteroids. Clin Exp Rheumatol 1995; 13: 293-7
50. Wolfe AM. The epidemiology of rheumatoid arthritis: a review. Bull Rheum Dis 1968; 19: 518-28
51. Chuang TY, Hunder GG, Ilstrup DM, et al. Polymyalgia rheumatica: a 10 yr epidemiologic and clinical study. Ann Intern Med 1982; 97: 672-7
52. Spector TD, Hall GM, McCloskey EV, et al. Risk of vertebral fracture in women with rheumatoid arthirits. BMJ 1993; 306: 558-68
53. Cooper CC, Wickham C. Rheumatoid arthritis, corticosteroid therapy and hip fracture. In: Christiansen C, Overgaard K, editors. Osteoporosis. Copenhagen: Osteopress, 1990
54. Laan RFJM, Bujjs WCAM, Verbeek ALM, et al. Bone mineral density in patients with recent onset of rheumatoid arthritis: influence of disease activity and functional capacity. Ann Rheum Dis 1993; 52: 21-6
55. Dykman TR, Gluck OS, Murphy WA, et al. Evaluation of factors associated with glucocorticoid induced osteopenia in patients with rheumatic diseases. Arthritis Rheum 1985; 28: 361-81
56. Hall GM, Spector TD, Griffin JA, et al. The effect of rheumatoid arthritis and steroid therapy on bone density in postmenopausal women. Arthritis Rheum 1993; 36: 1510-6
57. Manning PJ, Evans MR, Reid IR. Normal bone density following cure of Cushing's syndrome. Clin Endocrinol 1992; 36: 229-54
58. Laan RF, van Riel PL, van de Putte LB, et al. Low-dose prednisone induces rapid reversible axial bone loss in patients with rheumatoid arthritis: a randomized, controlled study. Ann Intern Med 1993 Nov 15; 119 (10): 963-8
59. Adachi JD, Bessen WD, Brown J, et al. Intermittent etidronate to prevent corticosteroid induced osteoporosis. N Engl J Med 1997; 337: 382-7
60. Schnitzer TJ. Alendronate and glucocorticoid induced osteoporosis [abstract 1174]. Arthritis Rheum 1997; 40 (9 Suppl. 2)
61. Sambrook P, Birmingham J, Kelly P, et al. Prevention of corticosteroid induced osteoporosis. N Engl J Med 1993; 328: 1747-52
62. Gallacher SJ, Fenner JAK, Anderson K, et al. Intravenous pamidronate in the treatment of osteoporosis associated with corticosteroid dependent lung disease: an open pilot study. Thorax 1992; 47: 932-6
63. Mulder H, Struys A. Intermittent cyclical etidronate in the prevention of corticosteroid induced bone loss. Br J Rheum 1994; 33: 348-50
64. Diamond T, McGuigan L, Barbagallo S, et al. Cyclical etidronate plus ergocalciferol prevents glucocorticoid induced bone loss in postmenopausal women. Am J Med 1995; 98: 459-63
65. Grecu EO, Simmons R, Baylink DJ, et al. Effects of medroxyprogesterone on some parameters of calcium metabolism in patients with glucocorticoid induced osteoporosis. Bone Miner 1991; 13: 153-61
66. Lukert BP, Johnson BE, Robinson RG. Estrogen and progesterone replacement therapy reduces glucocorticoid induced bone loss. J Bone Miner Res 1992; 7: 1063-9
67. Buckley LM, Leib ES, Cartularo KS, et al. Calcium and vitamin D3 supplementation prevents bone loss in the spine secondary to low-dose corticosteroids in patients with rheumatoid arthritis: a randomized, double-blind, placebo-controlled trial. Ann Intern Med 1996 Dec 15; 125: 961-8
68. Healey JH, Paget SA, Williamsrusso P, et al. A randomized placebo-controlled trial of salmon calcitonin for bone loss in glucocorticoid-treated temporal arteritis and polymyalgia rheumatica. Calcif Tissue Int 1996; 58: 73-80

Correspondence: Dr *Clifford J. Rosen*, Maine Center for Osteoporosis Research and Education, 176 Mount Hope Avenue, Bangor, ME 04402, USA.
E-mail: crosen@maine.maine.edu

New Bisphosphonates in the Treatment of Bone Diseases

Davide Gatti and *Silvano Adami*

University Hospital of Valeggio, University of Verona, Verona, Italy

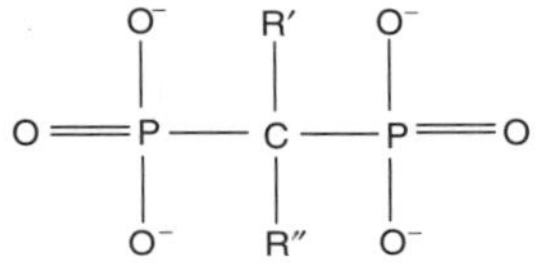

Fig. 1. Structure of germinal bisphosphonate.

Bisphosphonates are pyrophosphate analogues, in which the oxygen in P-O-P has been replaced by a carbon, resulting in a P-C-P structure. They are not a new class of agents and, in the past, were used exclusively as antiscaling agents. The activity of bisphosphonates in bone was discovered in the late 1960s but they became available for general use in human diseases of the bone only in the 1980s.[1,2] The bisphosphonates developed so far share a common strong anti-osteoclastic activity, and for these pharmacological properties they have been studied and nowadays are extensively used for the treatment of Paget's disease of bone, hypercalcaemia of malignancy, bone metastases, and several forms of osteoporosis. Despite important common features, the physicochemical and biological characteristics of the developed bisphosphonates may vary and should be considered individually with respect to both long term clinical use and toxicology.

The P-C-P bond together with the R′ (fig. 1) side chain provides the great affinity of bisphosphonates to the bone mineral.[1] The R″ side chain is responsible for the potency of the agents in inhibiting osteoclast activity.[3] The simplest R″ is a methyl in etidronate but it can be an aliphatic chain, a branched chain or a ring (fig. 2). The mechanism of action is not fully understood but it seems to differ substantially depending on the absence or presence of an NH_2 group.[4-6]

Bisphosphonates have become the treatment of choice for several diseases of interest in older patients. Their pharmacological characteristics, clinical use and tolerability profile have been recently reviewed.[2,7,8] In this review we will concentrate on the recent advances in understanding the mechanism of action, general pharmacology, and the clinical use of bisphosphonates, with particular attention on agents which have been only recently developed.

1. Pharmacology of Bisphosphonates

The intestinal absorption of bisphosphonates is low, ranging from 0.5 to 3%, and is abruptly decreased by the presence of food containing even a small amount of calcium salts. For this reason, they must be administered in strictly fasting conditions, with no food for at least 30 minutes after administration. Most of the bisphosphonate that enters into the circulation and remains unbound to protein is actively taken up by bone tissue and excreted in the urine with a clearance superior to that of the perfusion volume, indicating an active process of transport.[1,2,9] The skeletal uptake is about 50% of the dose of bisphosphonate absorbed, but this proportion may vary according to bone turnover and is not homogeneous; it is the highest at sites of active bone remodelling. These properties are why labelled bisphosphonates are used for bone scintiscan, and the reason for the extraordinary therapeutic activity of bisphosphonates in focal bone diseases such as Paget's disease or metastatic lesions.[9]

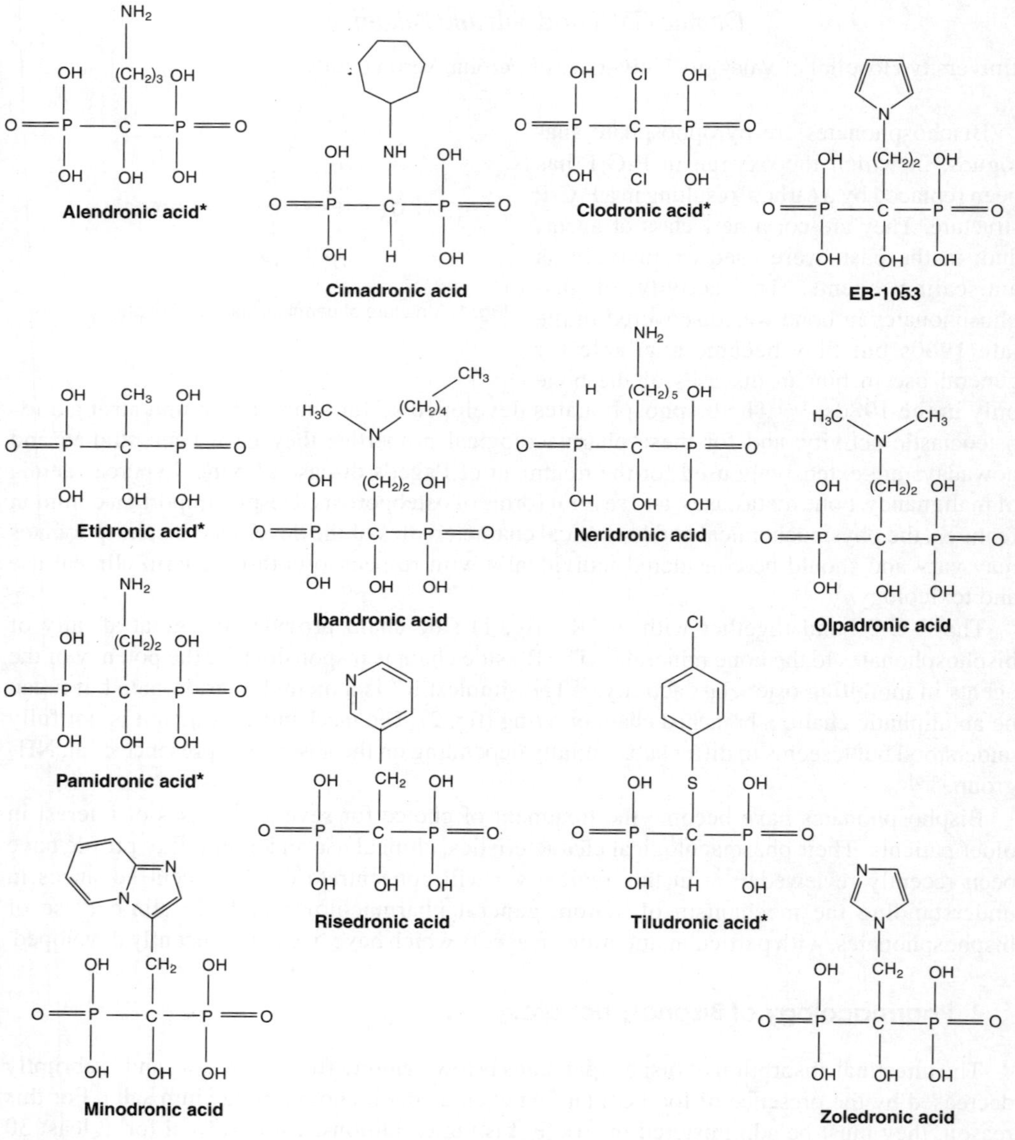

Alendronic acid*

Cimadronic acid

Clodronic acid*

EB-1053

Etidronic acid*

Ibandronic acid

Neridronic acid

Olpadronic acid

Pamidronic acid*

Risedronic acid

Tiludronic acid*

Minodronic acid

Zoledronic acid

Fig. 2. Chemical structures of bisphosphonates investigated for their skeletal effects in humans.
* = commercially available.

Bisphosphonates are released from the skeleton spontaneously at an extremely low rate, although it varies slightly for different agents according to their polarity. This difference in polarity explains the shorter terminal bone half-life of risedronate compared with neridronate or alendronate.

Most of the drug retained in the skeleton when initially administered is later released during skeletal remodelling. Thus, the amount of drug released which is likely to again become bioavailable depends on bone turnover: in humans it is in the order of a decade. However, the half-life of bisphosphonate activity is much shorter,[10] indicating that the bisphosphonate sequestered in bone is not pharmacologically active.

2. Mode of Action

The short circulating half-life of bisphosphonates minimises the exposure of non-target tissue, this is in addition to the effect of the generally high polarity on exposure. Thus, at the dosages usually recommended, the bisphosphonates concentrate at pharmacologically significant concentrations only at the bone surfaces and, in particular, inside the osteoclast which the bisphosphonates enter during the process of active bone resorption.[11,12]

A direct activity of the bisphosphonates on osteoclast activity has been shown both *in vitro* and *ex vivo*, leading to decreased formation, activity and life span of these cells. The decreased osteoclast recruitment seen with bisphosphonate therapy can be explained only by assuming an action on bone cells not lying on the bone surface or through an activity on other bone cells. Thus, the decreased osteoclast formation produced by bisphosphonates in tissue culture, has been attributed to a direct action on osteoblasts, which support osteoclast formation.[13]

It has been well documented that the entry of bisphosphonates in to osteoclasts during active bone reabsorption is associated with a rapid interruption of the resorbing activity with the disappearance of the convoluted membrane.[11,14]

The molecular mechanism of action of bisphosphonates on osteoclasts has been at least in part elucidated. Clodronate and possibly other compounds which do not contain an aminogroup, impair the synthesis of ATP with subsequent death of the cells. The aminobisphosphonates are responsible for bone apoptosis triggered by the inhibition of squalene syntheses and other enzymes involved in cholesterol metabolism. Interestingly, mevastatin mimics the effect of alendronate on osteoclast formation and the action of both is inhibited by mevalonic acid.[4,6]

These differences in molecular mechanism of action might explain why (at bone histomorphometry), in patients given aminobisphosphonates, inactive osteoclasts can be detected floating above the bone surfaces whereas the bone exposed to clodronate has a reduced number of bone cells.[15] It is not clear to what extent this difference in osteoclast survival may affect the long term outcome of therapy of Paget's disease or osteoporosis.

3. Tolerability Profile of Bisphosphonates

Bisphosphonates are generally well tolerated, but tolerability may vary considerably from one agent to another. Very high doses of etidronate impair the normal skeletal mineralisation and may even increase fracture incidence,[16] but at the doses used for the treatment of osteoporosis, no bisphosphonates induce clinical or histological signs of impaired mineralisation.[17,18]

The mechanical properties of the skeleton of animals treated over long periods with relatively high doses of various bisphosphonates have been shown to be perfectly preserved.[8] The experience in humans goes up to 7 years with the same encouraging tolerability profile for bone quality.[19]

When high intravenous doses of aminobisphosphonates (containing an NH group) are given to patients who have never received bisphosphonate therapy, particularly when parathyroid hormone (PTH) levels are not suppressed, the patients may experience fevers for 1 to 3 days associated with transient haematological changes resembling a typical acute-phase response.[20,21] High intravenous doses of aminobisphosphonates have been also associated with the appearance of ocular reactions.[8]

Because of the high renal clearance of all bisphosphonates, the concentration at the renal tubule easily reaches toxic levels during rapid intravenous infusions. These are strongly related with the amount of agent infused per unit time and it is strongly recommended to not exceed, at least for clodronate, an intravenous infusion rate of 200 mg/hour or 5 mg/min.[8] The infusion rate considered safe for pamidronate is 1 to 2 mg/min. For the most powerful bisphosphonates, such as ibandronate, the highest recommended intravenous dose is 2mg. This dose can be administered as an intravenous bolus, avoiding the need for unpractical low infusion rates, and making the treatment of osteoporosis with 2 to 4 bolus injections per year of a bisphosphonate an interesting alternative to continuous oral therapy.

Oral aminobisphosphonates may induce serious gastrointestinal lesions, with the sporadic appearance of erosive oesophagitis which is the result of the contact of undissolved crystals with the oesophageal or gastric mucosa. Increasing the speed of dissolution by the ingestion of the tablet with a large amount of water[22] and remaining in the upright position for 30 minutes after administration, can lessen these adverse events. Theoretically, however, less polar amino-compounds can be better tolerated, whereas the same does not appear to be true for the more powerful agents even with the lower amount of drug actually taken. In fact, the general impression is that the stronger the antiosteoclastic activity of the aminobisphosphonate, the higher their irritating effect on the mucosa.

4. Therapeutic Use of Bisphosphonates

4.1 Osteoporosis

Osteoporosis is a systemic skeletal disease characterised by a low bone mass and reduced bone strength which leads to increased risk of low trauma fractures.

Approximately 45% of White women at the age of 50 years will sustain an osteoporotic fracture over their remaining lifetime.[23] Hip fracture is a typical osteoporosis-related fracture responsible for excess mortality and long term disability in a large proportion of elderly people. Vertebral fractures may involve up to 30% of women above the sixth decade of life and are responsible for a sharp decline in the quality of life.[24] Even though bone mass is not the only determinant of fracture risk, it is by far the most important. It has been estimated that for any 10% decrease from the peak bone mass the risk of fracture rises by a factor of 2 to 3.[25] Bone losses of any type are invariably related to an uncoupling between bone resorption and bone formation. The bone loss associated with estrogen deficiency is related to increased bone turnover which increases the so called 'remodelling space' accounting for the 10% loss of bone mass occurring in the first 5 years after menopause.[26] Both mechanisms of bone loss can be corrected by bisphosphonate therapy which decreases bone turnover to premenopausal levels and blunts the reabsorbing activity of osteoclasts, thus apparently correcting the imbalance with osteoblastic bone formation.

Etidronate was the first bisphosphonate extensively studied for the treatment of osteoporosis. At high doses this agent impairs bone mineralisation and so it is usual to adopt an intermittent regimen (400 mg/day, 2 hours after a meal, for 2 weeks in a 3-month cycle). This administration regimen, which might be considered suboptimal, was nevertheless shown to prevent postmenopausal bone loss[27,28] and corticosteroid-induced osteoporosis,[29] and to increase bone mass in involutional osteoporosis.[30] Spinal bone density increased by about 4% within the first 2 years and then plateaued. A significant trend towards fracture risk reduction was shown in 2 studies after 2 years of follow-up,[29,31] but this effect was not significant at the completion of the third year. This is mainly as a result of the inadequacies relating to the study population rather than the effects of etidronate on bone mass.

To date, the most extensive and exhaustive studies on osteoporosis treatment have been with alendronate. Oral alendronate 5 to 10 mg/day at least 30 minutes before breakfast for 3 years has been shown to prevent postmenopausal bone loss and to increase spine and femoral neck bone mineral density by 8.8 and 5.9%, respectively, relative to placebo.[32] The dosages adopted in the Fracture Intervention Trial (FIT)[32] were either 5 or 10 mg/day or a mixture of these doses. However the optimal effect on bone mass was invariably associated with the 10mg dosage, which should be the initial recommended dose when the inevitable incomplete compliance with long term therapies is considered. The densitometric changes were accompanied by a halving of the incidence of patients with new vertebral deformities and femoral neck fracture.

The FIT trial included also 4432 women with osteopenia (femoral neck T score <1.6) without prevalent vertebral fracture. In this cohort of patients the treatment over 4 years significantly decreased the vertebral fracture incidence by 44%, but had no effect on non-vertebral fractures. Not surprisingly, the more pronounced effect on fracture was observed in the patients with osteoporosis (T score <2.5).[33] This should be intuitively attributed to the larger relative burden in patients without osteoporosis of fractures secondary to severe traumas. For the same reason the antifracture efficacy is greater in the patients with the highest risk of non-traumatic osteoporotic fractures. Interestingly, the effects on fracture risk were that predicted by the changes in BMD, as it appears from the results of prospective epidemiological studies[25] relating BMD to hip fracture risk. In a subanalysis of the FIT trial, Hockberg et al.[34] found that fracture incidence was related to both baseline BMD and its percentage changes during alendronate therapy, suggesting that among women taking bisphosphonates there is a proportionality between the increases in BMD and the risk reduction in new vertebral fracture.

Subanalysis of the FIT study showed that in postmenopausal women with pre-existing vertebral fracture, alendronate therapy for 3 years reduced the number of days of bed confinement and days of limited activity caused by back pain.[35] This further emphasises the relationship between the incidence of vertebral fracture and its effect on quality of life.

The combination of treatment with alendronate 10 mg/day and conjugated estrogens (0.625 mg/day) has been evaluated in two separate studies. This regimen produced larger increases in BMD than either agent alone and, above all, was not associated with adverse effects on bone mineralisation or bone fragility.[36,37]

In a study that included 1258 postmenopausal patients, the efficacy and safety of treatment with oral once-weekly alendronate 70mg, twice-weekly alendronate 35mg and daily alendronate 10mg were found to be comparable, suggesting the possibility of a once-weekly dosage regimen that might be considered more convenient for most patients.[38]

In the first large controlled trial on male osteoporosis therapy, alendronate was shown to increase both spine and hip BMD to an extent similar to that obtained with the same dosage in postmenopausal osteoporosis, and irrespective of the presence of hypogonadism.[39]

Alendronate was shown in a large-scale study to be highly effective for the prevention and treatment of glucocorticoid-induced osteoporosis.[40]

Tiludronate has been tested in osteoporosis in phase II studies,[41] but when the selected dosages were tested for the prevention of osteoporotic fractures they appeared inadequate and this led to interruption of the development of tiludronate for osteoporosis therapy.

4.2 New Compounds for Osteoporosis

A large clinical development programme with the aminobisphosphonate risedronate for osteoporosis therapy has recently been completed. In a study of the prevention of early postmenopausal bone loss,[42] oral risedronate 5mg fully prevented the bone loss observed in the patients treated with placebo with a mean percent difference (risedronate minus placebo) after 2 years of 5.5 and 3% for lumbar spine and femoral neck, respectively. In a year of post-treatment follow-up, bone loss was accelerated and the difference with the placebo group fell to approximately 3.2 and 2% for lumbar spine and femoral neck, respectively. This acceleration of bone loss was also observed with alendronate in a similar prevention study,[43] but was not observed when the same drug was given for the treatment of osteoporosis, despite a rapid resumption of bone turnover.[44,45] In a group of patients receiving oral risedronate 5mg cyclically (2 weeks of every calendar month), the bone loss preventing capacity was half that observed with continuous therapy with the same daily dose, indicating that 5 mg/day might not yet be the maximum effective dosage. In a prevention study[46] in women with artificially-induced menopause for breast cancer receiving oral risedronate 30 mg/day for 2 out of 12 weeks, the BMD changes were similar to those reported by Mortensen et al.[42] Interestingly, this intermittent dosage regimen is equal to 5 mg/day in terms of cumulative dosage. This lends support to the general belief that over a relatively long time interval (2 to 6 months) the effects on bone mass are related to the cumulative dose rather than the daily dose of bisphosphonate and provides the rationale for the results obtained with intermittent parenteral bisphosphonates.

To determine the efficacy and safety of risedronate in the prevention of vertebral fractures in postmenopausal women with established osteoporosis, two studies were conducted: one in North America (2458 patients)[47] and one in Europe and Australia (1226 patients).[48] Postmenopausal women with at least two radiographically confirmed vertebral fractures (European-Australian Study) or at least one vertebral fracture and low lumbar spine (American Study) received risedronate 2.5 or 5 mg/day or placebo. The duration of the studies was 3 years; however, the 2.5mg group was discontinued after 1 (American Study) and 2 (European-Australian Study) years, because of other data[49] showing that the 5mg dose produced a more consistent effect in increasing BMD while having a similar safety profile to the 2.5mg dose. There were significant differences in spine and hip BMD between the risedronate 5mg and control groups after 6 months. At 3 years treatment differences ranged from +4.3 to +5.9% at the spine and from +2.8 to +3.1 % at the femoral neck. Over 3 years the relative risk of new vertebral fracture in the risedronate 5mg group ranged from 0. 51 (0.36-0.73; European-Australian Study) to 0.59 (0.43-0.82; American Study), while the relative risk of nonvertebral fractures ranged from 0.6 (0.39-0.94) to 0.67 (0.44-1.04), respectively.

In the first controlled trial specifically designed to evaluate the effectiveness of an anti-resorptive drug in preventing hip fracture,[50] women with very low femoral neck bone mineral density (<–4 T score) or aged >80 years with a bone mass independent risk factor for hip fracture (most often risk of falling) were investigated. Overall 9337 patients were randomly assigned to receive risedronate (2.5 or 5mg daily) or placebo orally for 3 years, along with calcium (1000 mg/day) or vitamin D (up to 500 IU daily) if the serum 25-hydroxy-vitamin D level was low. Risedronate treatment significantly reduced the risk of hip fracture by 24% in the overall population (3.0% versus 4.0%, $p = 0.05$). In patients with low BMD hip fracture incidence was reduced by 39% and in those with prevalent fracture by 58%. In elderly patients (aged >80 years) with a clinical risk of hip fracture and unknown BMD values but who were likely to have a T score >–3, risedronate therapy had no effect, despite a high incidence of events (4.6% versus 5.1%). This suggests that elderly subjects with a high risk of falling do not substantially benefit from antiresorptive therapy if femoral neck BMD is relatively preserved.

The efficacy of risedronate therapy over 12 months was also studied in men and women on treatment for several conditions with moderate to high doses of corticosteroids (≥7.5mg of prednisone equivalent) within previous 3 months (prevention study).[51] or for more than 6 months (treatment study).[52] The two studies included 224 and 290 patients, respectively, who were randomised to receive either risedronate (2.5 or 5mg) or placebo. The percentage lumbar spine BMD changes relative to control patients ranged from 1.5 to 3.4, with the largest relative increases in the prevention study with the 5 mg/day dosage. In the two studies, 18 of 112 patients in the placebo group and 12 of 200 patients given either dose of risedronate experienced new vertebral fractures, with a highly significant 67% reduction in vertebral fracture risk relative to placebo. Of note is the high incidence of vertebral fracture in control patients despite treatment with 500 or 1000mg calcium supplements in the prevention and treatment studies, respectively. As in the study by Saag et al.,[40] most vertebral fractures occurred in postmenopausal women and in males.

The use of intermittent intravenous bisphosphonates has been pioneered by studies with alendronate, pamidronate and clodronate.[53-55] This treatment regimen has been chosen for an extensive clinical development for ibandronate. In phase II studies, this agent administered as an intravenous bolus (0.25, 0.5, 1 or 2mg) every 3 months for a year, resulted in BMD increases ranging from 2.4 to 5.2% and from 1.19 to 2.92% for lumbar spine and total hip, respectively.[56] Similar results were observed after administration of oral ibandronate 0.25 to 5mg once daily.[57] This indirectly suggests an oral bioavailability for ibandronate of 0.5 to 1%.

A clinical trial in 2862 postmenopausal women with at least one vertebral fracture given either placebo or ibandronate 0.5 or 1mg by intravenous injection every 3 months over 3 years has been recently completed.[58] The decrease in fracture rate in ibandronate-treated patients was not significant. The most obvious criticism of this study and the most obvious explanation for the disappointing results of this trial is the inadequacy of the dose and the selection of the patients, a large proportion of whom had spine BMD T scores just below –2. In such patients prevalent vertebral fractures are likely to have been traumatic and do not reflect a high risk of new events. This was particularly true in the North American arm of the study, where the overall number of vertebral fracture events was substantially lower than expected.

Other bisphosphonates [zoledronate, minodronate (YH-529)] are under the early phases of development for use in osteoporosis.

4.3 Paget's Disease

Paget's disease of the bone is a focal bone disease, characterised by an uncontrolled increase in bone remodelling with concomitant loss of the lamellar structure. The progression of the disease leads to the appearance at the involved skeletal segment of patchy lytic lesions alternating with sclerotic areas, bone hypertrophy and gross deformities. Disease may be confined to one bone or be widespread, and it occurs mostly in the pelvis, vertebrae, long bones and skull. At a microscopic level, increased bone turnover appears to result from an increase in the number of osteoclasts which are also abnormal in dimension, the number of nuclei, and the size of the individual reabsorption cavities.[59]

Calcitonin has been used to effectively suppress the excess osteoclastic activity, but this therapy has been abandoned in favour of bisphosphonates for the early relapses after discontinuation and for frequent resistance.[60] Bisphosphonates are currently regarded as practically the only treatment for Paget's disease. Etidronate was the first bisphosphonate shown to be affective in reversing the biochemical alteration of the disease, and also providing symptomatic relief. At the conventional dosages of 5 to 10 mg/kg/day over 3 to 6 months, 70% of the patients will respond with alkaline phosphatase levels falling to normal.[61] However the higher dosages (20 mg/kg/day) which might be required for controlling more severe disease cannot be recommended because of their adverse effect on bone mineralisation and renal phosphate retention.[62]

In an increasing number of countries, pamidronate and clodronate are also used for the treatment of Paget's disease.[63,64] These compounds administered intravenously, give better response rates relative to etidronate particularly in the most severe disease. The dose and the duration of bisphosphonate therapy should be tailored to the severity of the disease. The daily intravenous dose is usually 30 to 60mg for pamidronate and 300mg for clodronate over 5 to 14 days. The treatment course should aim to lower bone turnover to the midpoint of the reference range. In the treatment follow-up of Paget's disease, bone turnover can be assessed a few days after the treatment course using a marker of bone resorption, such as hydroxyproline or deoxypyridoline urinary excretion, but it is usually measured 6 months later using a marker for bone formation such as alkaline phosphatase.[65]

When adequate doses are used, treatment with bisphosphonates decreases markers of bone turnover to within the normal range. This cannot be apparently achieved in a small proportion of patients with widespread disease. In these patients, relapse of the disease occurs more rapidly and retreatment lowers bone turnover to the same nadir obtained with the previous treatment course. This apparent resistance can be managed in a proportion of patients by using very high intravenous doses of bisphosphonates,[66] but some patients appear to have true resistance with an unsuppressible component of the disease, the pathophysiology of which is unknown.

4.4 New Bisphosphonates for Paget's Disease

In the last year, a few new bisphosphonates, other than etidronate, clodronate and pamidronate, became available in several countries for the treatment of Paget's disease. Tiludronate,[67-69] alendronate[70-73] and risedronate[74-76] at oral dosages of 400, 40 and 30 mg/day, respectively, for 3 to 6 months have been shown to be superior to etidronate 400 mg/day. The mean decrease in excess bone turnover markers (i.e. difference between the patient marker and midpoint of normal range) was around 80% for all 3 agents, and the proportion of patients in whom serum alkaline phosphatase normalised within 6 months after commencing therapy was similar (60 to 70%). These 3 agents will provide an alternative to etidronate which may be abandoned in some countries because of its narrow therapeutic index in the treatment of Paget's disease.

The new bisphosphonates, tiludronate, alendronate and risedronate, have not been compared with each other or with other parenteral bisphosphonates. Any comparison is also made difficult by the different administration regimens adopted: 0.5 to 2 hours before breakfast for alendronate 10 and 40mg, 2 hours after a meal for etidronate and tiludronate. In fact, these differences might be associated with changes in the rate of intestinal absorption of 1- to 3-fold. The clinical success of these agents is likely to be related to their tolerability profile with special regard to the gastrointestinal tolerability. Ibandronate,[77] zoledronate[78,79] and alendronate[80,81] have been tested in some preliminary studies in Paget's disease using intravenous administration, and they are in later phase clinical trials for registration. The total intravenous doses of these agents needed to achieve the normalisation of serum alkaline phosphatase in more than 70% of the patients, are likely to be in the range of 40, 10 and 5mg for alendronate, ibandronate and zoledronate, respectively. These agents may provide a better alternative to parenteral clodronate and pamidronate if they can be administered as a bolus injection, rather than by slow intravenous infusions, with an acceptable tolerability profile.

4.5 Bone Metastases and Malignant Hypercalcaemia

Bone involvement is particularly common in patients with malignancy. Localised bone metastases are mostly seen in patients with breast or prostate cancer.[82,83] In other malignancies (e.g. neck, lung and kidney cancer, and multiple myeloma), the bone destruction is generalised and mediated by osteolytic factors, especially PTH-related protein (PTHrP), which is also able to act on the kidney by promoting tubular reabsorption of calcium.[84] In these malignancies, hypercalcaemia may appear early during tumour growth, whereas in patients with only bone metastases it is a late or even terminal complication associated with the tumour burden.[85]

Tumour cells can directly destroy bone, but in most cases they release local factors which activate osteoclastic activity.[86] It has been shown that even in the osteosclerotic lesions, the growth of the metastases inside bone tissue is preceded by the osteoclastic reabsorption of normal bone tissue.[87,88]

Where hypercalcaemia results only from local bone destruction within bone metastatic lesions, bisphosphonates are the treatment of choice. They provide rapid and persistent normalisation of hypercalcaemia, lessening of the growth of bone metastases, and some relief of bone pain, which represents often the principal concern of conservative therapy. Because the bisphosphonates are able to act exclusively on osteoclasts, it is not surprising that their efficacy is only partial and very transient when hypercalcaemia results from the production of systemic factors or when non-osteolytic mechanisms, such as increased renal tubular reabsorption of calcium, dehydration or decreased bone formation, are predominant.[89]

The great majority of studies in malignancy were carried out with pamidronate (intravenously) and clodronate (intravenously or orally). The intravenous route is usually preferred for the treatment of hypercalcaemia, which should be considered an acute condition. The usual dosage of clodronate is 300mg dissolved in 500ml of saline solution per day over 3 to 5 days.[90-92] Pamidronate is somewhat more potent than clodronate and this permits the administration of a single dose of up to 90mg,[64] which roughly corresponds in our experience to three 300mg clodronate infusions. This advantage is beneficial when hypercalcaemia tends to rapidly relapse and when frequent courses of treatment are needed.

The bisphosphonates have been also extensively tested in the prevention of 'bone events' (new metastases, fractures, episodes of hypercalcaemia) in patients with malignancy and the results have been considered encouraging. The dosages adopted are either oral clodronate (800 to 1200 mg/day)[93] or intravenous pamidronate (90mg every 4 weeks).[94] Recently, in an extensive trial in patients with breast cancer, long term treatment with clodronate 1600 mg/day significantly reduced the occurrence of new bone and nonskeletal metastases.[95] This later finding might suggest an affect of clodronate on the attachment of cancer cells to peripheral tissues.[96,97]

The bisphosphonates are also used for the symptomatic treatment of metastatic bone pain, even when the lesions are osteoblastic.[98,99] The dosages used are in general higher than for other indications and need to be tailored to individual patients.

4.6 New Bisphosphonates in Malignancy

Three studies with an intravenous formulation of ibandronate have been conducted in patients with hypercalcaemia of malignancy. Doses of ibandronate ranged from 0.2 to 2mg (30 patients),[100] 2 to 6mg (125 patients)[101] or 0.6 to 2mg (151 patients).[102] The duration of therapy was one or two single doses. Ibandronate reduced albumin-corrected serum calcium levels in all patients and the response was dose related. Normalisation of serum calcium was achieved in approximately 50% of the patients given ibandronate ≤2mg, and by 70% of the patients given ibandronate 4 to 6mg. The median time to relapse was 18 days for the patients in the 2 and 4mg dose groups and 26 days for the 6mg dose group. In the patients with initially higher PTHrP levels, serum calcium levels decreased to a lesser extent and the duration of the effect was also lower than in the patients with normal PTHrP levels at baseline.[103] A better response rate was observed in patients with breast and haematological tumours, and in the patients with moderate hypercalcaemia (<3.5 mmol/L).[101,102]

Zoledronate has been tested in a phase I trial in patients with tumour-induced hypercalcaemia. With a single intravenous infusion of 1.2 or 2.4mg, normal serum calcium levels were obtained in 19 of 20 patients and the median duration of action was 33 days.[104]

Incadronate has been tested in a few patients with hypercalcaemia of malignancy and the effective dose appears to be in the range of 1 to 2mg given as a single dose.[105]

Clinical studies examining the efficacy of ibandronate in patients with bone metastases did not address specific end-points such as bone pain or skeletal complications. Both a single intravenous bolus of ibandronate 3mg[106] or oral ibandronate (5 to 50 mg/day for 4 months)[107] were associated with significant decreases in the biochemical markers of bone resorption.

In 28 patients with carcinoma of the prostate metastatic to the skeleton, intravenous olpadronate 4mg daily for 5 days followed by oral olpadronate 200mg daily decreased bone pain in 76% of the patients and the clinical response paralleled the biochemical changes in bone resorption.[99]

5. Conclusions

The bisphosphonates are the treatment of choice for Paget's disease and hypercalcaemia of malignancy. In these conditions, the newer bisphosphonates may offer a wider range of options regarding method and frequency of administration. In terms of efficacy, they have all been shown to be superior to etidronate, whereas the advantage of any new agent over the others is uncertain. The results of recent clinical trials are likely to increase the use of bisphosphonates for the prevention of secondary bone lesions in patients with breast carcinoma or multiple myeloma.

An impressive amount of data has documented the efficacy of etidronate and even more particularly of alendronate and risedronate for the treatment of postmenopausal and corticosteroid-induced osteoporosis.

An impressive amount of data has documented the efficacy of etidronate and, even more, of alendronate for the treatment of postmenopausal and corticosteroid-induced osteoporosis. Data will be shortly available for risedronate and other bisphosphonates in these indications. These data are rapidly changing the clinical approach towards the prevention and treatment of osteoporosis, which is no longer regarded as an inevitable age-related disease.

References

1. Fleish H. Bisphosphonates: mechanism of action and clinical use. In: Mundy GR, Martin TJ, editors. Physiology and pharmacology of bone: handbook of experimental pharmacology. New York: Springer-Verlag, 1993: 377-418
2. Fleish H. Bisphosphonates: mechanism of action and clinical use. In: Bilezikian JP, Raisz LG, Rodan GA, editors. Principles of bone biology. San Diego: Academic Press, 1996: 1037-52
3. Geddes AD, D'Souza SM, Ebetino FH, et al. Bisphosphonates: structure activity relationship and therapeutic implications. J Bone Miner Res 1994; 8: 265-306
4. Luckman SP, Hughes DE, Coxon FP, et al. Nitrogen-containing bisphosphonates inhibit the mevalonate pathway and prevent post-translational prenylation of GTP-binding proteins, including rats. J Bone Miner Res 1998; 13: 581-9
5. Frith JC, Monkkonen J, Blackburn GM, et al. Clodronate and liposome-encapsualted clodronate are metabolized to atoxis ATP analog, adenosine 5′-beta,gamma-dichloromethylene triphosphate, by mammalian cells in vitro. J Bone Miner Res 1997; 12: 1358-67
6. Hughes DE, Wright KR, Uy HL, et al. Bisphosphonates promote apoptosis in murine osteoclasts in vitro and in vivo. J Bone Miner Res 1995; 10: 1478-87
7. Johansen A, Stone M, Rawlinson F. Bisphosphonates and the treatment of bone disease in the elderly. Drug Aging 1996; 8 (2): 113-26
8. Adami S, Zamberlan N. Adverse effects of bisphosphonates. Drug Saf 1996; 14 (3): 158-70
9. Papapoulos SE. Pharmacodynamics of bisphosphonates in man: implication for treatment. In: Bijovet OLM, Fleish H, Canfield RE, et al., editors. Bisphosphonate on bones. Amsterdam: Elsevier, 1995: 231-63
10. Adami S, Zamberlan N, Mian M, et al. Duration of the effects of intravenous alendronate in postmenopausal women and in patients with primary hyperparathyroidism. Bone Miner 1994; 25: 75-82
11. Sato M, Grasser W, Naoto E, et al. Bisphosphonate action: alendronate localization in rat bone and effects on osteoclasts culture. J Clin Invest 1991; 88: 2095-105
12. Masarachia P, Weinreb M, Balena R, et al. Comparison of the distribution of 3H-alendronate and 3H-etidronate in rat and mouse bones. Bone 1996; 19: 281-90
13. Sahni M, Guenther HL, Fleisch H, et al. Bisphosphonates act on rat bone resorption trough the mediation of osteoblasts. J Clin Invest 1993; 91: 2004-11
14. Sato M, Grasser W. Effects of bisphosphonates on isolated rat osteoclasts as examined by reflected light microscopy. J Bone Miner Res 1990; 5: 31-40
15. Boonekamp PM, van der Wee-Pals LJA, van Wijk-van Lennep MM, et al. Two modes of action of bisphosphonates on osteoclastic resorption of mineralized matrix. Bone Miner 1986; 1: 27-39
16. Flora L, Hassing GS, Cloyd GG, et al. The long-term skeletal effects of EHDP in dogs. Metab Bone Dis Relat Res 1981; 4/5: 289-300

17. Storm T, Steiniche T, Thamsborg G, et al. Changes in bone histomorphometry after long-term treatment with intermittent, cyclic etidronate for postmenopausal osteoporosis. J Bone Miner Res 1993; 8 (2): 199-208
18. Ott SM, Woodson GC, Huffer WE, et al. Bone histomorphometric changes after cyclic therapy with phosphate and etidronate disodium in women with postmenopausal osteoporosis. J Clin Endocrinol Metab 1994; 78: 968-72
19. Miller PD, Watts NB, Licata AA, et al. Cyclical etidronate in the treatment of postmenopausal osteoporosis: efficacy and safety after seven years of treatment. Am J Med 1997; 103: 468-76
20. Adami S, Bhalla AK, Dorizzi R, et al. The acute-phase response after bisphosphonates administration. Calcif Tissue Int 1987; 41: 326-31
21. Schweitzer DH, Oostendorp-van der Ruit M, van de Pluijm G, et al. Interleukin-6 and the acute phase response during treatment of patients with Paget's disease with the nitrogen-containing bisphosphonate dimethylaminohydroxy propylidene bisphosphonate. J Bone Miner Res 1995; 6: 956-62
22. De Groen PC, Lubbe DF, Hirsh LJ, et al. Esophagitis associated with the use of alendronate. N Engl J Med 1996; 355 (14): 1016-21
23. Melton LJ, Chrischilles EA, Cooper C, et al. Perspective: how many women have osteoporosis. J Bone Miner Res 1992; 7: 1005-10
24. Chrischilles EA, Butler CD, Davis CS, et al. A model of lifetime osteoporosis impact. Arch Intern Med 1991; 151: 2026-32
25. Cummings S, Black D, Nevitt M, et al. Bone density at various sites for prediction of hip fractures. Lancet 1993; 341: 72-5
26. Adami S, Kanis JA. Assessment of involutional bone loss: methodological and conceptual problems. J Bone Miner Res 1995; 10: 511-7
27. Herd RJM, Balena R, Black LM, et al. The prevention of early postmenopausal bone loss by cyclic etidronate therapy; a 2-year, double-blind, placebo-controlled study. Am J Med 1997; 103: 92-9
28. Meunier PJ, Confavreux E, Tupinon I, et al. Prevention of early postmenopausal bone loss with cyclical etidronate therapy (a double-blind, placebo-controlled study and 1-year follow-up). J Clin Endocrinol Metab 1997; 82: 2784-91
29. Adachi JD, Bensen WG, Brown J, et al. Intermittent etidronate therapy to prevent corticosteroid-induced osteoporosis. N Engl J Med 1997; 337: 382-421
30. Watts NB, Harris ST, Genant HG, et al. Intermittent cyclical etidronate treatment of postmenopausal osteoporosis. N Engl J Med 1990; 323: 73-9
31. Storm T, Thamsborg G, Steiniche T, et al. Effect of intermittent cyclical etidronate therapy on bone mass and fracture rate in women with postmenopausal osteoporosis. N Engl J Med 1990; 322 (18): 1265-71
32. Black DM, Cummings SR, Karpf DB, et al. Randomised trial of effect of alendronate on risk of fracture in women with existing vertebral fractures: Fracture Intervention Trial Research Group. Lancet 1996; 348: 1535-41
33. Cummings SR, Black D, Thompson DE et al. Effect of Alendronate on risk of fracture in women with low bone density but without vertebral frcatures. JAMA 1998; 280: 2077-82
34. Hockberg MA, Ross PD, Black D et al. Larger increases in bone mineral density during alendronate therapy are associated with a lower risk of new vertebral fractures in women with postmenopausal osteoporosis. Arth Rheum 1999; 42: 1246-54
35. Nevitt MC, Thompson DE, Black DM et al. Effect of Alendronate on limited-activity days and bed-disability days caused by back pain in postmenopausal women with existing vertebral fractures. Ann Intern Med 2000; 160: 77-85
36. Lindsay R, Cosman C, Lobo RA, et al. Addition of alendronate to ongoing hormone replacement therapy in the treatment of osteoporosis: a randomized, controlled trial. J Clin Endocrinol Metab 1999; 84: 3076-81
37. Bone HG, Greenspan SL, McKeever C et al. Alendronate and estrogen effects in postmenopausal women with low bone mineral density. J Clin Endocrinol Metab 2000; 85: 720-6
38 Schnitzer T, Bone HG, Crepaldi G. et al. Therapeutic equivalence of alendronate 70 mg once-weekly and alendronate 10 mg daily in the treatment of osteoporosis. Aging Clin Exp Res. Submitted for publication
39 Orwoll E, Ettinger M, Weiss S et al. Alendronate treatement of osteoporosis in men. N Engl J Med. In press
40. Saag KG, Emkey R, Schnitzer TJ, et al. Alendronate for the prevention and treatment of glucocorticoid-induced osteoporosis: the Glucocorticoid-Induced Osteoporosis Intervention Study Group. N Engl J Med 1998; 339 (5): 292-9
41. Reginster JY, Lecart MP, Deroisy R, et al. Prevention of postmenopausal bone loss by tiludronate. Lancet 1989; II: 1469-71
42. Mortensen L, Charles P, Bekker PJ, et al. Risedronate increases bone mass in an early postmenopausal population: two years of treatment plus one year of follow up. J Clin Endocrinol Metab 1998; 83 (2): 396-402
43. McClung M, Clemmesen B, Daifotis A. Alendronate prevents postmenopausal bone loss in women without osteoporosis. Ann Intern Med 1998; 128 (4): 253-61
44. Rossini M, Gatti D, Zamberlan N, et al. Long-term effects of a treatment course with oral alendronate of postmenopausal osteoporosis. J Bone Miner Res 1994; 11: 1833-7
45. Stock JL, Bell NH, Chesnut III CH, et al. Increments in bone mineral density of the lumbar spine and hip and suppression of bone turnover are maintained after discontinuation of alendronate in postmenopausal women. Am J Med 1997; 103: 291-7
46. Delmas PD, Balena R, Confravreux E. Bisphosphonate risedronate prevents bone loss in women with artificial menopause due to chemotherapy of breast cancer; a double-blind placebo controlled study. J Clin Oncol 1997; 15 (3): 955-62
47. Harris ST, Watts NB, Genant HK, et al. Effects of risedronate treatment on vertebral and non vertebral fractures in women with postmenopausal osteoporosis, a randomised controlled study. JAMA 1999; 282 (14); 1344-52
48. Reginster JY, Minne HW, Sorensen OH, et al. Randomized trial of the effect of risedronate on vertebral fractures in women with established postmenopausal osteoporosis. Osteoporos Int 2000; 11; 83-91
49. Fogelman I, Ribot C, Smith R, et al. Risedronate reverses bone loss in postmenopausal women with low bone mass: results from a multinational, double-blind, placebo-controlled trial. J Clin Endocrinol Metab 2000; 85: 1895-1900

50. McClung M, Eastell R, Bensen W, et al. Risedronate reduces hip fracture risk in elderly women with osteoporosis. Osteoporos Int 2000; 11 Suppl 2: S207
51. Cohen S, Levy RM, Keller M, et al. Risedronate therapy prevents corticosteroid-induced bone loss. Arth Rheum 1999; 42: 2309-18
52. Reid DM, Hughes RA, Laan RFJM, et al. Efficacy and safety of daily risedrionate in the treatment of corticosteroid-induced osteoporosis in men and women: a randomized trial. J Bone Min Res 2000; 15: 1006-13
53. Passeri M, Baroni MC, Pedrazzoni M, et al Intermittent treatment with intravenous 4-amino-1-hydroxybutylidene-1,1-bisphosphonate (AHButBP) in the therapy of postmenopausal osteoporosis. Bone Miner 1991; 15: 237-48
54. Thiébaud D, Burckardt P, Melchior J, et al. Two years effectiveness of intravenous pamidronate (APD) versus oral fluoride for osteoporosis occurring in the menopause. Osteoporosis Int 1994; 4: 76-83
55. Filipponi P, Pedretti M, Fedeli L, et al. Cyclical clodronate is effective in preventing postmenopausal bone loss: a comparative study with transcutaneous hormone replacement therapy. J Bone Miner Res 1995; 10: 697-703
56. Thiébaud D, Burckhardt P, Kriegbaum H, et al. Three monthly intravenous injections of ibandronate in the treatment of postmenopausal osteoporosis. Am J Med 1997; 103: 298-307
57. Ravn P, Clemmensen B, Riis BJ, et al. The effect on bone mass and bone markers of different doses of ibandronate: a new bisphosphonate for prevention and treatment of postmenopausal osteoporosis: a 1-year, randomized, double-blind, placebo controlled dose finding study. Bone 1996; 19 (10): 527-33
58. Recker RR, Stakkestad JA, Felsenberfg D, et al. A new treatment paradigm: quarterly injections of ibandronate reduce the risk of fractures in women with postmenopausal osteoporosis: results of a 3-year trial. Osteoporos Int 2000; 11 Suppl 2: S209
59. Singer FR, Roodman GD. Paget's disease of bone. In: Bilezikian JP, Raisz LG, Rodan GA, editors. Principles of bone biology. San Diego (CA): Academic Press, 1996: 969-77
60. Patel S, Lyons AR, Hosking DJ. Drugs used in the treatment of metabolic bone disease: clinical pharmacology and therapeutic use. Drugs 1993; 46 (4): 594-617
61. Dunn CJ, Fitton A, Sorkin EM. Etidronic acid: a review of its pharmacological properties and therapeutic efficacy in resorptive bone disease. Drug Aging 1994; 5: 446-74
62. Gibbs CJ, Aaron JE, Peacock M. Osteomalacia in Paget's disease treated with short-term, high dose sodium etidronate. BMJ 1986; 292: 1227-9
63. Kanis JA, McCloskey EV. The use of clodronate in disorders of calcium and skeletal metabolism. In: Kanis JA, editors. Calcium metabolism: progress in basic and clinical pharmacology. Basel: Karger, 1990; 4: 89-136
64. Fitton A, McTavish D. Pamidronate: a review of its pharmacological properties and therapeutic efficacy in resorptive bone disease. Drugs 1991; 41: 289-318
65. Papapoulos SE, Frölich M. Prediction of the outcome of treatment of Paget's disease of bone with bisphosphonates from short term changes in the rate of bone resorption. J Clin Endocrinol Metab 1996; 81 (11): 3993-7
66. Cundy T, Wattie D, King AR. High dose pamidronate in the management of resistant Paget's disease. Calcif Tissue Int 1996; 58: 6-8
67. McClung MR, Tou CKP, Goldstein NH, et al. Tiludronate therapy for Paget's disease of bone. Bone 1995; 17 Suppl.: 493S-6
68. Roux C, Gennari C, Farrerons J, et al. Comparative prospective, double blind, multicenter study of the efficacy of tiludronate and etidronate in the treatment of Paget's bone disease of bone. Arthritis Rheum 1995; 6: 851-8
69. Devogelaer JP, Malghem J, Stasse P, et al. Biological and radiological responses to oral etidronate and tiludronate in Paget's disease of bone. Bone 1997; 20 (3): 259-61
70. Adami S, Mian M, Gatti D, et al. Effects of two oral doses of alendronate in the treatment of Paget's disease of bone. Bone 1994; 15: 415-7
71. Siris E, Weinstein RS, Altman R, et al. Comparative study of alendronate versus etidronate for the treatment of Paget's bone disease of bone. J Clin Endocrinol Metab 1996; 81: 961-7
72. Reid IR, Nicholson GC, Weinstein RS, et al. Biochemical and radiological improvement in Paget's disease of bone treated with alendronate: a randomized placebo controlled trial. Am J Med 1996; 101 (4): 341-8
73. Khan SA, Vasikaran S, McCloskey EV, et al. Alendronate in the treatment of Paget's disease of bone. Bone 1997; 20 (3): 263-71
74. Singer FR, Clemens TL, Rachelle AE, et al. Risedronate, a highly effective oral agent in the treatment of patients with severe Paget's disease. J Clin Endocrinol Metab 1998; 83 (6): 1906-10
75. Hosking DJ, Eusebio RA, Chines AA. Paget's disease of bone: reduction of disease activity with oral risedronate. Bone 1998; 22 (1): 51-5
76. Siris ES, Chines AA, Altman RD, et al. Risedronate in the treatment of Paget's disease of bone: an open label, multicenter study. J Bone Miner Res 1998; 13 (6): 1032-8
77. Grauer A, Knaus J, Seibel M, et al. Treatment of Paget's disease of bone with the new bisphosphonates BM 21.0955 by intravenous bolus injection. J Bone Miner Res 1994; 9 Suppl. 1: S430
78. Arden-Cardone M, Siris ES, Lyles KW, et al. Antiresorptive effect of a single infusion of microgram quantities of zoledronate in Paget's disease of bone. Calcif Tissue Int 1997; 60: 415-8
79. Garnero P, Gineyts E, Schaffer AV, et al. Measurement of urinary excretion of non-isomerized and beta-isomerized forms of type I collagen breakdown products to monitor the effects of the bisphosphonate zoledronate in Paget's disease. Arthritis Rheum 1998; 41 (2): 354-60
80. Adami S, Salvagno G, Guerrera G, et al. Treatment of Paget's disease of bone with intravenous 4-amino-1-hydroxybuthylidene-1,1-bisphosphonate. Calcif Tissue Int 1986; 39: 226-9

81. O'Doherty DP, McCloskey EV, Vasikaran S, et al. The effects of intravenous alendronate in Paget's disease of bone. J Bone Miner Res 1995; 10: 1094-100
82. Rubens RD. Bone involvement in solid tumors. In: Bijvoet OLM, Fleisch HA, Canfield RE, et al., editors. Bisphosphonate on bones. Amsterdam: Elsevier, 1995: 337-47
83. Mundy GR, Martin TJ. Pathophysiology of skeletal complications of cancer. In: Mundy GR, Martin TJ, editors. Physiology and pharmacology of bone: handbook of experimental pharmacology. New York: Springer-Verlag, 1993: 641-71
84. Martin TJ, Moseley JM, Gillespie MT. Parathyroid hormone-related protein: biochemistry and molecular biology. Crit Rev Biochem Mol Biol 1991; 26: 377-95
85. Mundy GR, Guise TA. Hypercalcemia of malignancy. Am J Med 1997; 103: 134-45
86. Yoneda T. Mechanisms of preferential metastases of breast cancer to bone. Int J Oncol 1996; 9: 103-9
87. Urwin GH, Persival RC, Harris S, et al. Generalized increase in bone resorption in carcinoma of the prostate. Br J Urol 1985; 57: 721-3
88. Goltzman D. Mechanisms of development of osteoblastic metastases. Cancer 1997; 80 Suppl.: 1581-7
89. Walls J, Ratcliffe WA, Howell A, et al. Response to intravenous bisphosphonate therapy in hypercalcaemic patients with and without bone metastases: the role of parathyroid hormone-related protein. Br J Cancer 1994; 70: 169-72
90. Bonjour JP, Philippe J, Guelpa G, et al. Bone and renal components in hypercalcemia of malignancy and responses to a single infusion of clodronate. Bone 1988; 9: 123-30
91. Adami S. Bisphosphonates in prostate carcinoma. Cancer 1997; Suppl. 80: 1674-9
92. Plosker GL, Goa KL. Clodronate: a review of its pharmacological properties and therapeutic efficacy in resorptive bone disease. Drugs 1994; 47: 945-82
93. Kanis JA, Powles T, Paterson AHG, et al. Clodronate decreases the frequency of skeletal metastases in women with breast cancer. Bone 1996; 19 (6): 663-67
94. Hortobagyi GN, Theriault RL, Porter L, et al. Efficacy of pamidronate in reducing skeletal complications in patients with breast cancer and lytic bone metastases. N Engl J Med 1996; 335: 1785-91
95. Diel IJ, Solomayer EF, Costa S, et al. Reduction in new metastases in breast cancer with adjuvant clodronate treatment. N Engl J Med 1998; 339: 357-63
96. Van der Pluijm G, Vloedgraven H, van Beek E, et al. Bisphosphonates inhibit the adhesion of breast cancer cells to bone matrices in vitro. J Clin Invest 1996; 98: 698-705
97. Boissier S, Magnetto S, Frapport L, et al. Bisphosphonates inhibit prostate and breast carcinoma cell adhesion to unmineralized bone extracellular matrices. Cancer Res 1997; 57: 3890-4
98. Adami S, Mian M. Clodronate therapy of metastatic bone disease in patients with prostatic carcinoma. Recent Results Cancer Res 1989; 116: 67-72
99. Pelger RCM, Hamdy NAT, Zwinderman AH, et al. Effect of the bisphosphonate olpadronate in patients with carcinoma of the prostate metastatic to the skeleton. Bone 1998; 22 (4): 403-8
100. Wüster C, Shöter KH, Thiébaud D, et al. Methyl-pentylamino-propylidene-bisphosphonate (BM 21.0955): a new potent and safe bisphosphonate for the treatment of cancer-associated hypercalcemia. Bone Miner 1993; 22: 77-85
101. Ralston SH, Thiébaud D, Herrmann Z, et al. Dose-response study of ibandronate in the treatment of cancer-associated hypercalcemia. Br J Cancer 1997; 75 (2): 295-300
102. Pecherstorfer M, Ludwig H, Schlosser K, et al. Administration of the bisphosphonate ibandronate (BM 21.0955) by intravenous bolus injection. J Bone Miner Res 1996; 11: 587-93
103. Blind E, Rave F, Meinel T, et al. Levels of parathyroid hormone-related protein (PTHrP) in hypercalcemia of malignancy are not lowered by treatment with the bisphosphonate BM 21.0955. Horm Metab Res 1993; 25: 40-4
104. Body JJ. Clinical research update: zoledronate. Cancer 1997; 80 Suppl.: 1699-701
105. Usui T, Oiso Y, Tomita A, et al. Pharmacokinetics of icandronate, a new bisphosphonate, in healthy volunteers and patients with malignancy-associated hypercalcemia. Int J Clin Pharmacol Ther 1997; 35 (6): 239-44
106. Pecherstorfer M, Herrmann Z, Body JJ, et al. Randomized phase II trial comparing different doses of the bisphosphonate ibandronate in the treatment of hypercalcemia of malignancy. J Clin Oncol 1996; 14 (1): 268-76
107. Coleman RE, Purohit OP, Black C, et al. Ibandronate: a well-tolerated new oral bisphosphonate for the treatment of bone metastases [abstract]. Breast 1995; 4: 236

Correspondence: Dr *Silvano Adami*, University Hospital of Valeggio, University of Verona, 37067 Valeggio S/M, Verona, Italy.
E-mail: adami@borgoroma.univr.it

The Bone-Building Action of the Parathyroid Hormone

Implications for the Treatment of Osteoporosis

James F. Whitfield, Paul Morley and *Gordon E. Willick*

Institute for Biological Sciences, National Research Council of Canada, Ottawa, Ontario, Canada

People in the world's 7 major pharmaceutical markets (the US, France, Germany, Italy, Spain, the UK and Japan) are living longer and with this longer life come diseases which are very difficult and expensive to understand and treat. Among these diseases is the fragile and spontaneous fracturing of bones of osteoporosis. The number of people with osteoporosis is increasing, and, with this, substantial long term demands on healthcare services and, thus, governments.[1-4] At the beginning of this century, osteoporosis was not the problem it is today. Then, the few patients with osteoporosis could be ignored without economic or political fallout, whereas now they have the political clout needed to force governments and healthcare professionals to do something about their failing skeletons.

Until the 1990s the best that could be done for a person with osteoporosis was to slow or stop their bone loss. There was no drug to strongly and directly stimulate bone growth to replace the lost bone, or to greatly increase the amount of remaining bone. However, the situation is changing fast. The first of today's most promising family of bone-building drugs was discovered 68 years ago,[5-7] but its osteogenic action was ignored or not believed until very recently. This family of drugs includes the native parathyroid hormone (PTH), PTH-(1-84), and several of its variously bioactive fragments. Until recently, PTH was believed only to inhibit phosphate uptake and stimulate Ca^{++} uptake by kidney tubule cells, and to cause bone resorption. However, now we know that it can strongly stimulate bone growth when administered in a certain way. Here we can only briefly summarise what is known about the osteogenicity of PTHs in animals and humans, but the interested reader should consult some of the more comprehensive reviews and collections of reviews to get the full detailed story of the PTHs and their potential for treating osteoporosis.[4,8-10]

1. What Causes Osteoporosis?

Both men and women can develop osteoporosis. In fact 20% of people with osteoporosis are men. However, because most people with osteoporosis are women, we will focus on what happens to the bones of women after menopause.

Although the bones of men also steadily weaken with age as testosterone levels gradually decline and this can ultimately lead to 'low-turnover' type II osteoporosis by around age 75 years, the precipitous menopausal estrogen crash in women triggers a 4- to 8-year acceleration of cortical thinning and cracking and even greater trabecular perforation and loss.[3,4] (It must be noted that the bones of a man also need the autocrine/paracrine estrogen, 17ß-estradiol, metabolised from gradually declining testosterone levels by aromatase found in osteoblasts to maintain bone mass.)[11-13] The effect on a woman of this accelerated bone loss depends on the peak bone mass when she is around 30 years of age. Bone mineral density (BMD) may decrease by 1 standard deviation below the average peak value into a 'pseudo-osteoporotic' osteopenic state in which fragile bones are still able to withstand the muscular strains imposed on them by the usually less strenuous daily activities of an elderly person without breaking, but they are more vulnerable to breakage by falls (elderly women fall more often than elderly men) and other accidents.[14] However, the accelerated loss may decrease the BMD more than 2.5 standard deviations below the peak value and into a true type I osteoporotic state in which the hip and wrist, but particularly the vertebrae, become so fragile that they can be broken or crushed even by the muscular strains imposed on them by normal daily movements.[14]

To understand that loss, we must first understand how bone is maintained. Bone needs continuous micromaintenance in the mature skeleton. The agents of this micromaintenance are the basic multi-cellular units (BMUs) first identified by Frost.[15] A BMU starts out as a team of osteoclasts collecting on a specifically signalling area of bone.[15,16,16a] The osteoclasts then remove that area releasing a large amount of Ca^{++} from the bone mineral, matrix collgen I breakdown products and a host of growth factors, such as bone morphogenetic protein (BMP)-2, insulin-like growth factors [IGF-I, IGF-II, IGF binding protein-5 (IGFBP-5)], and transforming growth factor (TGF)β, which had been locked in the bone by the osteoblasts of the previous BMU.[4,16] However, it is uncertain how many of these protein factors can survive the proteases from the osteoclasts.

At this point, the BMU shifts into formation phase. The osteoclasts without PTH receptors are replaced by mature, 'plump', PTH receptor-expressing, bone-building osteoblasts. The osteoblasts are recruited, attracted, and stimulated to mature by factors such as endothelin-1 from the endothelial cells of invading capillary loops[16b] and perhaps from receptors activated by the surviving factors liberated by the osteoclasts from the bone and then supplemented at the appropriate stage by the signals from integrin receptors activated by adhesion to extracellular matrix components such as the freshly deposited collagen I. Added to these are signals from Ca^{++} receptors (CaRs) on the osteoblasts (which are similar to parathyroid cell CaRs) activated by the released Ca^{++}. It seems that this Ca^{++} cloud is a key part of the mechanism that limits bone resorption and couples resorption to formation because while stimulating the CaRs on osteoblasts, it also activates the CaRs on the osteoclasts that released it and, thereby, inactivates them.[17-19] This resorption terminating, coupling function of the osteoclast and osteoblast CaRs is supported by data showing that the oral administration of NPS 2143, a specific CaR blocker, increased bone resorption in ovariectomised (OVX) rats.[20]

The osteoclast inactivation is followed by the activation of the osteoblast-driven excavation-refilling phase of the BMU. However, the osteoblasts of BMUs on the endosteal and trabecular surfaces do not completely refill the holes and trenches whereas the periosteal (cambial) osteoblasts tend to overfill the holes.[21-23] Consequently, over the years, endosteal and trabecular bone disappears and cortical shells thin. As a result of these changes, the overall diameters of weight-bearing bones such as the femoral shaft increase which compensates to some extent for the overall bone loss by increasing the bones' resistance to bending and hence breaking.[24] However, in one very important site, the femoral neck, there is no periosteum which means that the diameter of the neck does not increase with age. The combination of the thinning cortical shell and the loss of the internal trabecular supports without a compensatory increase in diameter makes the neck especially vulnerable to bending and breaking.[23,24]

At any moment, millions of BMUs are at work repairing and remodelling about 10% of the skeleton with holes to be filled that together make up the so-called 'remodelling space'.[3,21-23,25] By derepressing osteoclast recruitment and activity, the estrogen crash increases the rate of BMU activation and, thus, the bone turnover rate.[21,22,26] However, there is also an increasing preference of stromal stem cell progeny to develop into adipocytes rather than osteoblasts which translates into smaller teams of osteoblasts for formation-phase BMUs and slower refilling of excavations.[22,26] Since it normally takes as long as 3 to 4 months for osteoblasts in formation-phase BMUs to replace the bone demolished by osteoclasts in just 2 to 3 weeks, the combination of an increasing number of osteoclast teams and smaller osteoblast teams results in an exponentially escalating bone loss.[27] Bones now more rapidly lose trabeculae, regional strains increase, micro-cracks spread as cortical bone becomes increasingly Swiss cheese-like, load-bearing ability drops, hips become more bendable and breakable, and height is lost as weakened vertebral bodies collapse.[27]

How might the estrogen crash increase BMU activation and bone loss? Fundamentally, the crash increases the osteoclast development rate and lowers the apoptotic death rate. It does this in many converging, although still very incompletely defined, ways. First, preosteoclasts have estrogen receptors, the activation of which by 17β-estradiol limits the size of the osteoclast population by causing the preosteoclasts to kill themselves by apoptosis.[28] Consequently, the estrogen crash would increase the preosteoclast lifespan and ultimately increase osteoclast production.[28] These longer-lived progenitors are in turn stimulated by an increased production of cytokines such as macrophage-colony stimulating factor (M-CSF), interleukin (IL)-1β and IL-1β-induced tumour necrosis factors (TNFs) by bone marrow monocytes.[29-31] The responsiveness of the osteoclast progenitors to the increased production of TNF-inducing IL-1β is enhanced by the disappearance of the non-signalling IL-1 type 2 'decoy' receptors on marrow cells and osteoclasts that were diverting IL-1β from its signalling-competent receptors before the crash.[31] The cytokines also increase the number of marrow stromal/osteoblast progenitors with RANK ligand (ODF, osteoclast differentiation factor) on their surfaces that drive osteoclast differentiation by activating RANK receptors on the surfaces of osteoclast progenitors clustering around them.[30] These osteoblastic marrow cells further enhance osteoclast differentiation and survival with a derepressed production of IL-6 and IL-11.[29,30] Yet another contributor to the increased osteoclast production and ultimately BMU activation may be a drop in the normally estrogen-dependent nitric oxide (NO) production to a level that promotes osteoclast generation instead of restraining it, as the higher pre-crash NO level did.[32,33]

However, the effects of estrogen loss are not restricted to increasing the population of longer-lived osteoclasts in the bone marrow. TGFß stores in the bone matrix also decrease.[29] This means that less TGFβ can be released by osteoclasts (if, of course, any of it survives the osteoclasts' proteases) to repress further osteoclast production and stimulate osteoclast apoptosis, and to stimulate the migration of immature osteoblasts into the excavation site.[29] There is increased apoptotic death of osteocytes which, because they are the bones' microdamage sensors, would impair damage detection and activation of repair mechanisms.[34] Osteoblast activities, such as matrix deposition and growth factor secretion, may be reduced and the BMU replacement deficit thereby increased without the Ca^{++} and cyclic adenosine monophosphate (cAMP) signals from the cells' non-genomic surface estrogen receptors.[35] Finally, although undoubtedly more will be found, is the perhaps surprising possibility that there may be a loss of the fraction of intestinal Ca^{++} uptake that is driven by signals from the non-genomic estrogen receptors on the surfaces of intestinal mucosal cells.[36,37]

The loss of bone in a woman with osteoporosis can be reduced or stopped, but not reversed, by estrogens or a partial estrogen-mimicking selective estrogen receptor modulator (SERM) such as raloxifene.[2,38] It can also be reduced or stopped by calcitonin which inhibits osteoclast formation and action.[30,39,40] Then there are the bisphosphonates, such as alendronate, pamidronate and tiludronate, which, when they are incorporated into the bone hydroxyapatite prevent osteoclast recruitment, prevent osteoclasts from differentiating and attaching to bone, and kill mature osteoclasts by causing them to trigger apoptosis.[41-43] These anti-osteoclast agents are known collectively as antiresorptives which have only a limited bone-building action resulting from the promptly reduced osteoclast activity and continuing osteoblast activity (temporary osteoblastic 'overshoot') that gives the osteoblasts of formation-phase BMUs a chance to refill at least part of the resorption spaces which account for about 10% of the total bone volume.[41,42]

2. Parathyroid Hormone (PTH), a Potent Bone-Builder

While it is obviously helpful to suppress osteoclasts and allow the existing holes in the bones of the patient with osteoporosis to be refilled, a truly osteogenic (anabolic) drug which can increase the size, activity and the working life of osteoblasts, and strengthen remaining bone and bypass local mechanostatic limits, would be better.[27] Just such an agent is the native PTH-(1-84), the osteogenic potency of which was first glimpsed by Bauer et al.[5] in 1929 and then clearly demonstrated 3 years later in rats by Hans Selye[7] in response to the observation by Bauer et al.[5] and the surprising suggestion by Péhu et al.[6] that the lethal osteopetrosis of an 8-year-old boy was the work of the PTH from his enlarged parathyroid glands.

The PTH holohormone is an 84-amino acid protein, the 'conventional' receptor (there is at least one other version) for which is a serpentine, 7-transmembrane domain molecule.[4,44,45] This 'conventional' receptor is known as type 1 PTH/parathyroid–hormone-related protein (PTHrP) receptor (or PTHR1 receptor) because it can be activated by either PTH or peptides containing the PTH-related 1-34 part of the 139-, 141-, or 173-amino acid PTHrP. All of the bioactive motifs of the hormone seem to be in the 1 to 34 part of the molecule. The hydrophobic surface of the hormone's large amphiphilic α-helix between residues 16 and 34 binds to the receptor's extracellular N terminal region between residues 99 and 177 and the hormone then inserts its N terminal residues into the clustered transmembrane α-helices.[4,44,45] This triggers configurational shifts in the two regions of the receptor molecule that expose the guanosine triphosphate (GTP)/guanosine diphosphate (GDP) exchanger sites that convert inactive GDP•$G_{\alpha s}$ and GDP•$G_{\alpha q}$ complexes to active GTP•$G_{\alpha s}$ and GTP•$G_{\alpha q}$ complexes.[4,44,45] These complexes respectively and independently activate adenylyl cyclase and phospholipase C-β1 (PLC-β1), and the 2 functions of the hormone are separable.[4,45] Thus, PTH fragments, such as 1-desamino-hPTH-(1-34), hPTH-(3-34), hPTH-(13-34) and hPTH-(8-84) bind to the receptor's 99-177 region and expose the GTP/GDP exchanger site for the PLC-β1-activating $G_{\alpha q}$ protein, but they cannot expose the $G_{\alpha s}$-specific exchanger site and activate adenylyl cyclase, because they do not have functional N termini.[4] On the other hand, the C terminally truncated hPTH-(1-31)NH_2 and [Leu^{27}]*cyclo*(Glu^{22}-Lys^{26})hPTH-(1-31)NH_2 can activate adenylyl cyclase, but not PLC-β1, as effectively as the larger PTHs in cells such as proximal mouse kidney tubule cells and ROS17/2 osteogenic rat osteosarcoma cells and fetal human osteoclasts.[46-48a] However, these mini-PTHs can stimulate PLC-β1 in certain other cells such as specifically engineered LLC-PK1 pig kidney cells with very large numbers of conventional receptors or spleen lymphocytes which express unconventional PTH receptors.[49,50]

It must be pointed out that the once seemingly simple understanding of PTH signalling is now fading fast. There is increasing awareness of the existence of more PTH receptors and at least 1 more effector, phospholipase-D.[46,51,52]

3. The Animal Experience

The main features of the osteogenic action of PTH have been established between 1932 and today by extensive experimentation on dogs, ferrets, monkeys and sheep, but mainly OVX rats.[4,8,9,53,54] These features are now so clearly defined that they can be concisely summarised in the following few paragraphs.

Injecting 1 small, optimally effective dose of the native hormone or one of its adenylyl cyclase-stimulating N terminal fragments [e.g. hPTH-(1-30)NH_2, hPTH-(1-31) NH_2, hPTH-(1-34)OH, [Leu^{27}]*cyclo* (Glu^{22}-Lys^{26})hPTH-(1-31)NH_2, hPTH-(1-35) NH_2, hPTH-(1-36) and hPTH-(1-38)OH], but not a fragment [e.g. hPTH-(8-84)] that only stimulates PLC-β1 and/or protein kinase-Cs, each day stops OVX-induced bone loss, stimulates cortical bone growth and increases trabecular thickness far above the baseline value. An example of this typical PTH action from our laboratory is given in figure 1. Although, resorption is also stimulated, it is overridden by the anabolic component (fig. 1). In contrast, continuously infusing the same or larger doses of one of these molecules overrides the anabolic component and results in bone resorption (fig. 2).

PTH is most potently osteogenic in fetal and newborn animals whose grow-

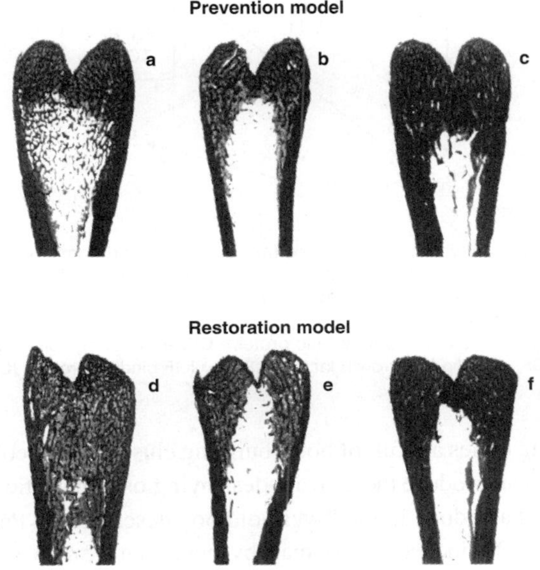

Fig. 1. Examples of how parathyroid hormones (PTHs), in this case, [Leu^{27}]*cyclo*(Glu^{22}-Lys^{26})hPTH-(1-31)NH_2 (ostabolin-C), prevent the loss of femoral trabeculae and greatly stimulate the growth of the trabeculae remaining after prolonged ovariectomy-induced estrogen deprivation. In the 'prevention' experiment 2 nmoles of the fragment/100g of bodyweight were injected subcutaneously once each day 6 days/week for 6 weeks starting 2 weeks after ovariectomy. As can be seen from these typical examples, the peptide (**c**) essentially stopped the very large ovariectomy-induced loss of trabeculae (**b**) in the distal femurs and increased the mean metaphyseal trabecular thickness to a value that was 3.3 times greater than the mean trabecular thickness in the sham-operated control rats (**a**). In the 'restoration' experiment the daily injections of the peptide started 9 weeks after ovariectomy and stopped 6 weeks later (**e**). Ostabolin-C stopped any further ovariectomy-induced trabecular loss between the 9th and 15th week, but it did not replace already lost trabeculae (**f**). However, the treatment dramatically increased the mean thickness of the remaining trabeculae (**f**) which was 3.2 times greater than the mean trabecular thickness in the control distal femurs (**d**). The distal femurs were decalcified, sectioned and stained exactly as described by Whitfield et al.[45] (**a**), (**d**): sham-operated; (**b**), (**e**): ovariectomy plus daily injections of acidic saline vehicle (0.15 mol/L NaCl in distilled water containing 0.001N HCl); (**c**), (**f**): ostabolin-C in acidic saline vehicle.

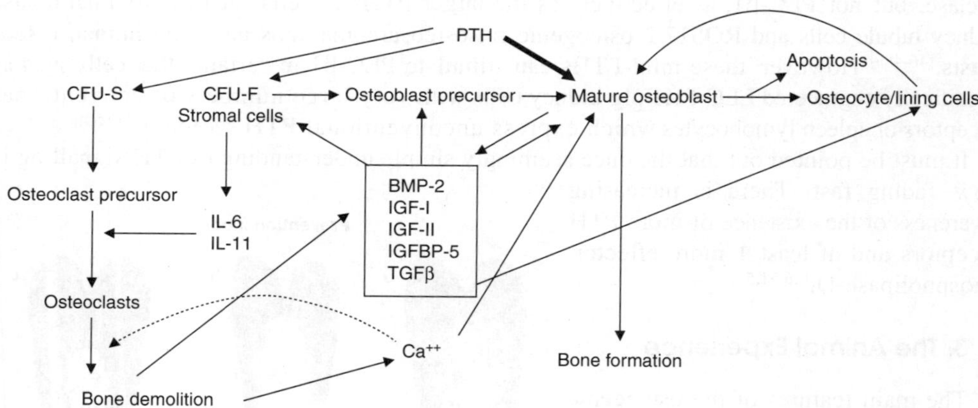

Fig. 2. A hypothetical scenario for how parathyroid hormone (PTH) can both build and demolish bone. If injected in small daily boluses, PTHs bone-building or anabolic action will predominate, but when injected in larger boluses or when continuously infused its bone-demolishing or catabolic action will predominate (reproduced from Whitfield et al.,[4] with permission).
BMP = bone morphogenetic protein; **CFU-F** = colony forming unit-fibroblast; **CFU-S** = colony forming unit-stem; **IGF** = insulin-like growth factor; **IGFBP** = IGF binding protein; **IL** = interleukin; **TGF** = transforming growth factor.

ing bones are full of bone-building clusters of osteoblasts covered with PTH receptors.[4,22,23,55] It can produce the marrow-destroying osteopetrotic bone growth in such animals as it appears to have done in the 8-year-old boy described by Péhu et al.[6,23]

PTH increases bone mass by increasing the number, activity and working lifespan of osteoblasts. The hormone or its fragments do not need prior BMU activation and osteoclast activity to maximally stimulate bone growth in the osteoblast-loaded skeletons of young growing rats, or in older animals with a high bone turnover and, thus, a large population of osteoblast-bearing formation-phase BMUs. However, it probably has to activate osteoclasts to get enough formation-phase BMUs and, thereby, enough PTH receptor-bearing osteoblasts to maximally stimulate bone growth in old animals with low bone turnover and few BMUs.

Neither PTH nor its adenylyl cyclase-stimulating fragments can generate new trabeculae nor can they stimulate the reconnection of trabeculae that have drifted too far apart (fig. 1).[4,53,54] In other words, they cannot replace trabeculae that have already been lost. However, they can reinforce existing trabecular connectivity and disproportionately increase bone strength by stimulating the layering of the remaining trabeculae and their connecting struts with osteoblasts depositing thick layers of normal lamellar bone.[53,54,56]

The new PTH-induced bone may be rapidly resorbed when the treatment stops because the OVX animal is still without osteoclast-suppressing estrogens and the increased new bone load may now exceed local mechanostatic set points.[27] This new bone can be protected from the osteoclasts by an antiresorptive agent such as alendronate, calcitonin, estrogen or raloxifene.

Finally, PTH can promote fracture healing. For example, daily injections of hPTH-(1-34) 200 μg/kg bodyweight increased ultimate bone load and callus volume of fractured mouse tibias by as much as 75 and 99%, respectively, over the control values 20 days after fracturing and 175 and 72%, respectively, over the control values 40 days after fracturing.[57]

4. An Osteogenic Scenario

How PTH or a PTH fragment might build bone is still far from known. Nevertheless all of the currently available information from the animal studies has been surveyed and woven into the hypothetical scheme of figure 2 which presents the mechanisms that are likely to be responsible for the paradoxical ability of PTH to both build and resorb bone.[4,56] According to this scheme, when PTH is injected subcutaneously as single daily doses it reaches target cells in both the bone and the bone marrow. In the bone marrow, it stimulates the proliferation of the pluripotent CFU-S (colony forming units-stem) haematopoietic stem cells in the bone marrow. This increases the population of macrophage/osteoclast precursors and ultimately the number of BMUs. It will also directly or indirectly stimulate marrow stromal cells which are either bipotential adipocyte/osteoblast precursors or already committed osteoblast progenitors.

The PTH-induced bursts of adenylyl cyclase activity may directly or indirectly stimulate the stromal osteoblast precursors to proliferate and make autocrine/paracrine agents such as IGFs and TGFß to stimulate themselves, their neighbours and osteoblast precursors in adjacent bone. Then the proliferatively active preosteoblasts make their way directly and/or via the blood to the bone where they join osteoblast teams in growing bones or the formation-phase BMUs in mature bone. While still immature and proliferatively active they make and deposit matrix components such as osteopontin and collagen I. But when the volume of signals from their collagen-activated integrin receptors reaches a certain level they turn off their cell cycle genes and turn up the PTHR1 receptor gene expression and then the genes for proteins such as osteocalcin that process and mineralise the matrix they had deposited while immature.

The stromal precursor cells will also make M-CSF as well as IL-6 and IL-11, which will induce the progeny of the PTH-stimulated CFU-S cells first to choose the macrophage option and then become osteoclasts. Thus, PTH, like an estrogen crash, increases BMU activation and with it bone resorption. However, the main targets of the first PTH dose, the 'first-response' cells, are the densely receptored mature osteoblasts of growing skeletons and the formation-phase BMUs of mature remodelling skeletons. Since these cells have shut off their cell cycle genes they won't proliferate in response to signals directly or indirectly triggered by PTH. Instead they produce autocrine and paracrine osteogenic mediators such as IGFs and TGFβ, as well as vascular endothelial cell growth factor to stimulate the formation of more blood vessels to feed the new bone. They also produce more connexin-43 to form gap junctions for a temporary intercellular 'osteo-internet' which connects them to their neighbours and other cells such as stromal precursor cells which do not have PTH receptors. This enables them to transmit the signals from their PTH receptors widely to bring a variety of precursor cells and bone-lining cells into the osteogenic response team. The signals flowing through this pathway and the various cytokines and other osteogenic factors released from the bone matrix by the osteoclasts also reversibly convert synthetically inactive bone-lining cells without PTH receptors into active osteoblasts covered with PTH receptors. These 'second-response' cells now start building bone and at the same time expand the 'osteo-internet' by reversibly converting their neighbouring lining cells into the next wave of PTH-responsive osteoblasts.

The net outcome of this spreading response to single daily PTH pulses is a growth of bone which, unlike the growth resulting from antiresorptive treatment, can override the limits imposed by local mechanostatic set-points.

However, when PTH is continuously infused or injected in super-optimal doses there is still a massive accumulation of mature osteoblasts which produce and secrete IGF-I and IGF-II. But they now, when stimulated by continuous PTH infusion, produce IGFBP-3, IGFBP–4 and mac25/IGFBP-7 which bind to, and thus inactivate, the IGFs.[58,59] Also under the continuous stimulation by PTH, osteoclasts produce cytokines such as IL-6, and osteoclast differentiation factor appears on the surface of marrow stromal/osteoblastic cells, both of which increase osteoclast production. PTH-stimulated osteoblasts also express the stem cell factor/steel factor (SCF or c-Kit ligand) and RANK ligand which stimulate osteoclast production by activating the Kit and RANK receptors on preosteoclasts.[30,60] The net outcome has switched from bone building to bone resorption.

5. The Human Experience

Expert opinion is that effective true anabolic agents for bone will be available by 2005 with PTH-like agents being among the most promising.[61] The extensive animal experience is undoubtedly largely responsible for this opinion. But what has been the human experience?

Despite the early indications of the potent osteogenicity of PTH, it took 45 years for this to be tested in postmenopausal women.[62,63] In the 1976 study of Reeve et al.,[62,63] 4 patients with osteoporosis received 100 μg/kg of hPTH-(1-34) fragment once daily by subcutaneous injection for 6 months and iliac trabecular bone growth was increased without a detectable effect on femoral BMD. In the next uncontrolled, multicentre study by the same group, 16 female and 5 male patients with osteoporosis receiving daily subcutaneous injections of hPTH-(1-34)OH 50 to 100 μg/kg for 6 to 24 months, had significantly increased iliac trabecular volume with new, normally mineralised lamellar bone.[64] Further tests have confirmed that PTH can stimulate the growth of bone, especially trabecular (cancellous) bone, in patients with osteoporosis with no significant short term adverse effects, and are discussed in this section.

5.1 Treatment Regimens

Although there have been many clinical studies of PTH as a drug for treating established osteoporosis, there is as yet no standard treatment protocol. The native hPTH-(1-84) and the hPTH-(1-38) fragment have been used, but it is hPTH-(1-34) that has been used most often. The doses used in these studies have been 25 to 40μg (400 to 600U) per day. The patients have been both men and women with osteoporosis with or without vertebral fractures. More recently, cyclic treatments have been used in which hPTH-(1-34) is injected subcutaneously for defined periods (e.g. once each day for 28 days) separated by relatively long treatment-free intervals (e.g. 3 months).

5.2 Bone Mineral Density and Fracture Incidence

The most commonly used end-point in clinical PTH trials has been BMD as measured by dual energy X-radiation absorptiometry (DEXA), quantitative computed tomography (QCT) and ultrasonography. Low BMD is closely correlated to increased fracture risk. Indeed, the fracture risk doubles for each standard deviation unit the BMD is below the mean peak BMD for people of the same gender.

In a 3-year study by Lindsay et al.,[65] hPTH-(1-34) 25 μg/day increased the vertebral BMD by 13% in 34 women with osteoporosis already receiving estrogen replacement therapy whereas the vertebral BMD did not change in the control group. This increased BMD was accompanied by reduced vertebral crushing as indicated by a 15% reduction in height loss. The increases were lower in bones with smaller trabecular fractions such as hip (2.7%) and forearm (1.0%). The overall total body BMD had increased by 8%. Hesch et al.[66] found a 20% increase in vertebral BMD after 14 months of hPTH-(1-38) 54 μg/day followed by nasal calcitonin in 13 women with osteoporosis.

In 30 women with osteoporosis receiving a 2-year cyclical treatment with hPTH-(1-34) [800U or 60μg per day for 28 days with 3-month rest periods],[67] there was a 10.2% increase in the lumbar vertebral BMD, a 2.4% increase in the femoral neck BMD and a 80% reduction in fracture incidence. This yearly increase of about 5% in spinal BMD is similar to increases induced by antiresorptive agents or fluoride.[67]

In a different kind of study, hPTH-(1-34) 40μg per day prevented the loss of vertebral bone caused by the estrogen crash triggered in 20 premenopausal women by the gonadotropic hormone-releasing hormone antagonist, nafarelin. However, there was no increase in the BMD.[68]

The results of the study by Neer et al.,[69] for a while cast doubt on PTH as a credible therapeutic agent for osteoporosis. They found that administering calcitriol (1′,25$(OH)_2$-vitamin D_3) and hPTH-(1-34) to 15 women with osteoporosis for 1 to 2 years increased lumbar vertebral BMD by 32%, but there was a net 4% reduction of the radial BMD. If true, this could have meant that while PTH would stop vertebral crushing it would increase the far more debilitating and dangerous hip fractures. To explain this they hypothesised that PTH had somehow 'stolen' cortical bone to make trabecular bone. However, this 'cortical steal' hypothesis has since been disproven. The common human experience is similar to the animal experience; PTH strongly stimulates trabecular bone growth and either does not affect or stimulates cortical bone growth.[70,71]

5.3 Histomorphometry

The trabecular bone in the iliac crests of women with osteoporosis responds like the femoral and tibial trabeculae of OVX rats to intermittent injections of a PTH fragment such as hPTH-(1-34).[70-74] Increased osteoid volumes, increased active surfaces and increased formation fronts, as revealed by sequential labelling with tetracycline, and a tendency for increased connectivity have all been shown with long term treatment. In addition, a 3-fold increase in formation rate was seen even after 2 years indicating that patients were still gaining bone.[74] The new bone was architecturally normal, normally mineralised, and trabecular widths and thicknesses had increased by as much as 25% above the baseline values. It has also been observed that the fragment [hPTH-(1-34)] can cause osteoblasts to start depositing new bone on surfaces which have not been pre-excavated by osteoclasts.[73] In other words PTH can stimulate the generation of osteoblasts in mature human skeletons without first activating osteoclasts and BMUs.

5.4 Serum Markers of Bone Formation

The principal serum markers for bone formation are osteocalcin, procollagen I C terminal peptides, and heat-labile alkaline phosphatase. Bone resorption markers are urinary hydroxyproline and pyridinoline/deoxypyridinoline, cross-linked N- and C- telopeptides of collagen I.

As expected, formation markers are consistently increased by intermittent PTH injections. For example, the daily hPTH-(1-34) injections in the study by Lindsay et al.[65] resulted in serum osteocalcin levels increasing for the first 6 months after which they slowly returned to baseline levels by 3 years. Cosman et al.[75] found that the daily hPTH-(1-34) injections that stimulated bone formation in women with osteoporosis in the study by Lindsay et al.[65] actually caused the serum osteocalcin and procollagen I C terminal peptide levels to rise during the first 4 to 6 weeks. Such an early serum osteocalcin surge signals a rapid build-up of mature osteoblasts.

As indicated in the scheme of figure 2, PTH also stimulates osteoclast generation and, thus, should also cause the appearance of the resorption markers. However, the changes in these markers caused by intermittent PTH injections are far less consistent than the changes in the formation markers. Urinary hydroxyproline has been found to increase, decrease or not change following PTH treatment.[71] While osteoblast-generated serum osteocalcin levels increased in the patients with osteoporosis in the study by Cosman et al.[75] during the first month of hPTH-(1-34) treatment, the osteoclast response, as indicated by the generation of cross-linked N-telopeptides, was delayed until 6 months and then returned to baseline values by 24 months.

5.5 PTH and Antiresorptive Therapy

The overall animal experience has shown that antiresorptives such as the SERM raloxifene can considerably reduce the dose of PTH needed to optimally stimulate bone growth in rats.[76] Although the PTH-induced bone is rapidly lost if the PTH injections are stopped, this can be prevented by continuing to administer the antiresorptive.[77] However, the use of the antiresorptive calcitonin by women with osteoporosis between periods of PTH treatments did not enhance the osteogenic response to PTH.[67] On the other hand, the use of nasal calcitonin after hPTH-(1-38) injections may have been responsible for the large (20%) increase in vertebral BMD in the patients of Hesch et al.[66] In addition, treatment with daily subcutaneous injections of recombinant hPTH-(1-84) 50 to 100μg for 1 year followed by oral alendronate 10 mg/day for 1 year, increased vertebral BMD by 12.5% which was much more than the increase observed with alendronate alone.[78]

Can co-treatment, as opposed to sequential treatment, with an antiresorptive agent affect PTH action? Of course the answer may depend on the availability of first-response osteoblasts. As expected, antiresorptive co-therapy does not blunt the osteogenic action of PTH in growing rats with their osteoblast-loaded skeletons. On the other hand, co-treatment with tiludronate blunts the osteogenicity of PTH in old ewes with low bone turnover.[79] In these animals, the osteoclast/BMU-activating action of PTH is required to produce enough osteoblasts via formation-phase BMUs for an optimal osteogenic response. So far, the limited experience with postmenopausal women, who probably had high levels of bone turnover, is that co-therapy with estrogen or the bisphosphonate alendronate did not reduce the osteogenic potency of hPTH-(1-34).[75] Therefore, the protection of new PTH-induced bone in such women with antiresorptives can be started during PTH treatment.

6. Future Osteogenic PTH Analogues

The next generation of osteogenic PTHs, the new mini-PTHs, have been invented and are now being tested in animals. Examples of these are hPTH-(1-31)NH_2 and the more potent [Leu^{27}]*cyclo*(Glu^{22}-Lys^{26})hPTH-(1-31)NH_2. They are the smallest of the potently osteogenic PTHs, although it must be noted that hPTH-(1-30)NH_2 is as osteogenic as the larger molecules at 25- to 50-fold higher doses in OVX rats.[80] Indeed, despite this very large dose required to stimulate bone growth in rats, hPTH-(1-30)NH_2 and its derivatives might turn out to be clinically useful because of the much greater sensitivity of humans to PTH.

The new mini-PTH-like molecules may be cheaper to produce than the larger PTH fragments, but most importantly they or their future derivatives may be deliverable orally or in aerosols. Some recent evidence from studies in mice and humans suggests that they may have the very important advantage of being effective anabolic agents with a much-reduced ability to stimulate bone resorption. Thus, hPTH-(1-31)NH_2 is as strong a stimulator of bone formation (as indicated by elevation of the serum osteocalcin levels) as hPTH-(1-34), but it is a much poorer stimulator of bone resorption than hPTH-(1-34) in several mouse strains.[81] In addition, hPTH-(1-31)NH_2 appears to be a much poorer stimulator of bone resorption than hPTH-(1-34) but it can stimulate adenylyl cyclase as effectively as hPTH-(1-34) in humans.[82] Another possible advantage of hPTH-(1-31)NH_2 and [Leu^{27}]*cyclo*(Glu^{22}-Lys^{26})hPTH-(1-31)NH_2 is their ability to stimulate adenylyl cyclase but not PLC-ß1 in normal mouse proximal convoluted kidney tubule cells and the osteogenic, but neoplastic, ROS17/2 osteosarcoma cells.[42-48] If this is also true for healthy, mature osteoblasts in human bone, it would be an important safety feature because PLC-activated protein kinase-Cs are strong, indeed the archetypal, tumour promoters.[83] Of course, both they and the large PTHs also have the advantage of being able to locally produce, and use as a mediator, the osteogenic IGF-I, which, if injected subcutaneously, could spread throughout the body and promote the growth of a variety of tumours especially in older people with nests of carcinogen-initiated cells in various organs such as the breast.[84]

7. Conclusion

It follows from both the extensive experience with animals, and the much more limited experience with men and women with osteoporosis, that PTH, or one of its adenylyl cyclase-stimulating fragments, will sooner or later be used to treat established osteoporosis by stimulating the formation of architecturally normal and biomechanically strong bone. The first generation hPTH-(1-84) and hPTH-(1-34) are currently in clinical trial and will be the first to reach the market. If they can survive the process of larger and better controlled clinical trials, PTH and its derivatives will be amongst the brightest stars on the clinical horizon for the growing number of people with osteoporosis.

References

1. Marchand G. Commercial exploitation of parathyroid hormone therapy for the treatment of postmenopausal osteoporosis. In: Whitfield JF, Morley P, editors. Anabolic treatments for osteoporosis. Boca Raton (FL): CRC Press, 1998: 175-83
2. Sannes LJ. Osteoporosis market set to expand with new drug launches. In: Decision Resources Spectrum Series. Spectrum: therapies markets and emerging technologies. Waltham: Decision Resources, 1998
3. Stevenson JC, Lindsay RL, editors. Osteoporosis. London: Chapman and Hall Medical, 1998
4. Whitfield JF, Morley P, Willick GE. The parathyroid hormone: an unexpected bone builder for treating osteoporosis. Austin (TX): Landes Bioscience, 1998

5. Bauer E, Aub JC, Albright F. Studies of calcium and phosphorus metabolism: V. a study of the bone trabeculae as a readily available reserve supply of calcium. J Exp Med 1929; 49: 145-62
6. Péhu M, Policard A, Dufort A. L'Ostéopetrose ou maladie des os marmoréens. Presse Med 1931; 53: 999-1003
7. Selye H. On the stimulation of new bone-formation with parathyroid extract and irradiated ergosterol. Endocrinology 1932; 16: 547-58
8. Dempster DW, Cosman F, Parisien M, et al. Anabolic action of parathyroid hormone. Endocr Rev 1993; 14: 690-709
9. Reeve J. PTH: a future role in the management of osteoporosis? J Bone Miner Res 1996; 11: 440-5
10. Whitfield JF, Morley P, editors. Anabolic treatments for osteoporosis. Boca Raton (FL): CRC Press, 1997
11. Morishima A, Grumbach MM, Simpson ER, et al. Aromatase deficiency in male and female siblings caused by a novel mutation and the physiological role of estrogens. J Clin Endocrinol Metab 1998; 80: 3689-98
12. Sharpe RM. The role oestrogen in the male. Trends Endocrinol Metab 1998; 9: 371-7
13. Vanderschueren D, Van Herck E, DeCoster R, et al. Aromatization of androgens is important for skeletal maintenance of aged male rats. Calcif Tissue Int 1996; 59: 179-83
14. World Health Organization (WHO). Assessment of fracture risk and its application to screening for osteoporosis [WHO Technical Report Series]. Geneva: WHO, 1994
15. Frost HM. Tetracycline-based histological analysis of bone remodelling. Calif Tissue Int 1969; 3: 211-37
16. Martin TJ, Dempster DW. Bone structure and cellular activity. In: Stevenson JC, Lindsay R, editors. Osteoporosis. London: Chapman and Hall Medical, 1997: 1-28
16a. Parfitt AM. Osteoclast precursors as leukocytes: importance of the area code. Bone 1998; 23: 491-4
16b. Parfitt AM. The mechanism of coupling. A role for the vasculature. Bone 2000; 26: 319-23
17. Kameda T, Mano H, Yamada Y, et al. Calcium-sensing receptors in mature osteoclasts which are bone-resorbing cells. Biochem Biophys Res Commun 1998; 245: 419-22
18. Baron R, Ravesloot J-H, Neff L, et al. Cell and molecular biology of the osteoclast. In: Noda M, editor. Cellular and molecular biology of bone. San Diego (CA): Academic Press, 1993: 445-95
19. Zaidi A, Adebanjo OA, Moonga BS, et al. Emerging insights into the role of calcium ions in osteoclast regulation. J Bone Miner Res 1999; 14: 669-74
20. Gowen M, Stroup GB, Bradbeer KN, et al. An antagonist of the parathyroid cell Ca^{2+} receptor stimulates PTH secretion and bone turnover in osteopenic ovariectomized rats [abstract]. Bone 1998; 23: S163
21. Eriksen EF, Axelrod DW, Melsen F. Bone histomorphometry. New York: Raven Press, 1994
22. Eriksen EF, Langdahl B, Klassen M. The cellular basis of osteoporosis. Spine: State Arts Revs 1994; 8: 23-62
23. Frost HM. Osteoporoses: their nature and therapeutic targets. In: Whitfield JF, Morley P, editors. Boca Raton (FL): CRC Press, 1998: 1-27
24. Einhorn TA. Biomechanics of bone. In: Bilezekian JP, Raisz LG, Rodan GA, editors. Principles of bone biology. San Diego (CA): Academic Press, 1996: 25-37
25. Hoyland JA, Neary J, Baris C, et al. Loss of osteocyte estrogen receptor expression in men with idiopathic osteoporosis [abstract]. Bone 1998; 22: 10S
26. Thomsen IS, Mosekilde L, Boyce RM, et al. Stochastic simulation of vertebral trabecular bone remodelling. Bone 1994; 15: 655-66
27. Dempster DW. Exploiting and bypassing the bone remodelling cycle to optimize the treatment of osteoporosis. J Bone Miner Res 1997; 12: 1152-4
28. Zecchi-Orlandini S, Formigli L, Tani A, et al. 17β-estradiol induces apoptosis in the proetseoclastic FLG 29.1 cell line. Biochem Biophys Res Commun 1999; 255: 680-5
29. Jilka RL. Cytokines, bone remodelling, and estrogen deficiency. Bone 1998; 23: 75-8
30. Hofbauer LC, Khoslab S, Dunstan CR, et al. The roles of osteoprotegerin ligand in the paracrine regulation of bone resorption. J Bone Miner Res 2000; 15: 2-12
31. Pilbeam C, Rao Y, Alander C, et al. Downregulation of mRNA expression for the 'decoy' interleukin-1 receptor 2 by ovariectomy. J Bone Miner Res 1997; 12 Suppl. 1: S433
32. Brandi ML, Hukkanen M, Umeda T, et al. Bidirectional regulation of osteoclast function by nitric oxide synthase isoforms. Proc Natl Acad Sci U S A 1995; 92: 2954-8
33. Holliday LS, Dean AD, Kin RH, et al. Low NO concentrations inhibit osteoclast formation in mouse marrow cultures by a cGMP-dependent mechanism. Am J Physiol 1997; 272 (3 Pt 2): F283-91
34. Tomkinson A, Gevers EF, Wit JM, et al. The role of estrogen in the control of rat osteocyte apoptosis. J Bone Miner Res 1998; 13: 1243-50
35. Nemere I, Farach-Carson MC. Membrane receptors for steroid hormones: a case for specific binding sites for vitamin D metabolites and estrogens. Biochem Biophys Res Commun 1998; 248: 443-9
36. Picotto G, Massheimer V, Boland R. Acute stimulation of intestinal calcium influx induced by 17β-estradiol via the cAMP messenger system. Mol Cell Endocrinol 1996; 119: 129-34
37. Salih MA, Sims SH, Kalu DN. Putative intestinal estrogen receptor: evidence for regional differences. Mol Cell Endocrinol 1996; 121: 47-55
38. Lindsay R. Estrogen and osteoporosis. In: Stevenson JC, Lindsay R, editors. London: Chapman and Hall Medical, 1998: 161-71
39. Roodman GD. Advances in bone biology: the osteoclast. Endocr Rev 1996; 17: 308-32
40. Shen Y, Li M, Wronski TJ. Calcitonin provides complete protection against cancellous bone loss in the femoral neck of ovariectomized rats. Calcif Tissue Int 1997; 60: 457-61
41. Fleisch H. Bisphosphonates in bone disease. New York: The Parthenon Publishing Group, 1997
42. Fleisch H. Bisphosphonates: mechanisms of action. Endocr Rev 1998; 19: 80-100

43. Hughes DE, Wright KE, Uy HL, et al. Bisphosphonates promote apoptosis in murine osteoclasts in vitro and in vivo. J Bone Miner Res 1995; 10: 1478-87
44. Bergwitz C, Gardella TJ, Flannery MR, et al. Full activation of chimeric receptors by hybrids between parathyroid hormone and calcitonin. J Biol Chem 1996; 271: 26469-72
45. Iida-Klein A, Guo J, Takemura M, et al. Mutations in the second cytoplasmic loop of the rat parathyroid hormone (PTH)/PTH-related protein receptor results in selective loss of PTH-stimulated phospholipase C activity. J Biol Chem 1997; 272: 6882-9
46. Friedman PA, Gesek FA, Morley P, et al. Cell-specific signalling and structure-activity relations of parathyroid hormone analogs in mouse kidney cells. Endocrinology 1999; 140: 301-9
47. Whitfield JF, Morley P, Willick G, et al. Stimulation of the growth of femoral trabecular bone in ovariectomized rats by the novel parathyroid hormone fragment hPTH-(1-31)NH_2 (ostabolin). Calcif Tissue Int 1996; 58: 81-7
48. Whitfield JF, Morley P, Willick G, et al. Cyclization by a specific lactam increases the ability of human parathyroid hormone hPTH-(1-31)NH_2 to stimulate bone growth in ovariectomized rats. J Bone Miner Res 1997; 12: 1246-52
48a. Wu Y, Kumar R. Parathyroid hormone regulates transforming growth factor β1 and β2 synthesis in osteoblasts via divergent signaling pathways. J Bone Miner Res 2000; 15: 879-84
49. Takasu H, Guo J, Bringhurst FR. Human and rat PTH/PTHrP display different signal selectivity for HPTH(1-31) and HPTH(1-30) in stably transformed LLC-PK1 cells [abstract]. J Bone Miner Res 1997; 12: S444
50. Whitfield JF, Isaacs RJ, MacLean S, et al. Stimulation of membrane-associated protein kinase-C activity in spleen lymphocytes by hPTH-(1-31)NH_2, its lactam derivative, [Leu^{27}]-cyclo(Glu^{22}-Lys^{26})-hPTH-(1-31)NH_2, and hPTH-(1-30)NH_2. Cell Signal 1999; 11: 159-64
51. Singh MKT, Kunnel JG, Strieleman PJ, et al. Parathyroid hormone (PTH)-(1-34), [$Nle^{8,18}$,Tyr^{34}]PTH-(3-34) amide, and PTH-related peptide –(1-34) stimulate phosphatidylcholine hydrolysis in UMR-106 osteoblastic cells: comparison with effects of phorbol 12,13-dibutyrate. Endocrinology 1999; 140: 131-7
52. Takasu H, Guo J, Bringhurst FR. Dual signaling and the ligand selectivity of the human PTH/PTHrP receptor. J Bone Miner Res 1999; 14: 11-20
53. Mosekilde L. Osteoporosis: mechanisms and models. In: Whitfield JF, Morley P, editors. Anabolic treatments for osteoporosis. Boca Raton (FL): CRC Press, 1998: 31-81
54. Wronski TJ, Li M. PTH: skeletal effects in the ovariectomized rat model for postmenopausal bone loss. In: Whitfield JF, Morley P, editors. Boca Raton (FL): CRC Press: 59-81
55. Walker D. The induction of osteopetrotic changes in hypophysectomized, thyroparathyroidectomized, and intact rats of various ages. Endocrinology 1971; 89: 1389-406
56. Whitfield JF, Morley P, Langille RM, et al. Adenylyl cyclase-activating anabolic agents: parathyroid hormone and prostaglandins E. In: Whitfield JF, Morley P, editors. Anabolic treatments for osteoporosis. Boca Raton (FL): CRC Press: 109-49
57. Andreassen TT, Ejersted C, Oxlund H. Intermittent parathyroid hormone (1-34) treatment increases callus formation and mechanical strength of healing rat fractures. J Bone Miner Res 1999; 14: 960-8
58. Pereira R, Canalis E. Parathyroid hormone induces mac25/ insulin-like growth factor binding protein 7 expression in osteoblasts [abstract]. Bone 1998; 23; S566
59. Watson PH, Fraher LJ, Kiesel D, et al. Enhanced osteoblast development after continuous infusion of rhPTH-(1-84) in the rat. Bone 1999; 24: 89-94
60. Blair HC, Julian BA, Cao X, et al. Parathyroid hormone-regulated production of stem cell factor in human osteoblasts and osteoblast-like cells. Biochem Biophys Res Commun 1999; 255: 778-84
61. Gruber HE, Farley SM, Baylink DJ. Predictions on future diagnosis and treatment of osteoporosis: results and discussion of a recent opinion poll. Calcif Tissue Int 1995; 57: 83-5
62. Reeve J, Hesp R, Williams D, et al. Anabolic effect of low doses of a fragment of human parathyroid hormone on the skeleton in postmenopausal osteoporosis. Lancet 1976; I: 1035-6
63. Reeve J, Tregear GW, Parsons JA. Preliminary trial of low doses of human parathyroid hormone fragment 1-34 in treatment of osteoporosis. Clin Endocrinol 1976; 21: 469-77
64. Reeve J, Meunier PJ, Parsons JA, et al. Anabolic effect of human parathyroid human fragment on trabecular bone in involutional osteoporosis: a multicenter trial. BMJ 1980; 280: 1340-4
65. Lindsay R, Nieves J, Formica C, et al. Randomised controlled study of effect of parathyroid hormone on vertebral bone mass and fracture incidence among postmenopausal women on oestrogen with osteoporosis. Lancet 1997; 350: 550-5
66. Hesch RD, Busch U, Prokop M, et al. Increase of vertebral density by combination therapy with pulsatile 1-38 PTH and sequential addition of calcitonin nasal spray in osteoporotic patients. Calcif Tissue Int 1989; 44: 176-80
67. Hodsman AB, Fraher LJ, Watson PH, et al. A randomized controlled trial to compare the efficacy of cyclical parathyroid hormone versus cyclical parathyroid hormone and sequential calcitonin to improve bone mass in post-menopausal women with osteoporosis. J Clin Endocrinol Metab 1997; 82: 620-8
68. Finkelstein JS, Klibanski A, Schafer EH, et al. Parathyroid hormone for the prevention of bone loss induced by estrogen deficiency. N Engl J Med 1994; 331: 1618-23
69. Neer R, Slovik D, Daly M, et al. Treatment of postmenopausal osteoporosis with daily parathyroid hormone plus calcitriol. In: Christiansen C, Overgaard K, editors. Osteoporosis. Copenhagen: Osteopress APS, 1991: 1314-7
70. Bradbeer JN, Arlot ME, Meunier PJ, et al. Treatment of osteoporosis with parathyroid peptide (hPTH-34) and oestrogen: increase in volume density of iliac cancellous bone may depend on reduced trabecular spacing as well as increased thickness of packets of newly formed bone. Clin Endocrinol 1997; 37: 282-9
71. Hodsman AB, Fraher LJ, Watson PH. Parathyroid hormone: the clinical experience and prospects. In: Whitfield JF, Morley P, editors. Anabolic treatments for osteoporosis. Boca Raton (FL): CRC Press, 1997: 83-1

72. Hodsman AB, Fraher LJ, Ostbye T, et al. An evaluation of several biochemical markers of bone formation and resorption in a protocol utilizing cyclical parathyroid hormone and calcitonin in therapy of osteoporosis. J Clin Invest 1993; 91: 1138-48
73. Hodsman AB, Steer BM. Early histomorphometric changes in response to parathyroid hormone therapy in osteoporosis: evidence for de novo bone formation on quiescent cancellous surfaces. Bone 1993; 14: 523-7
74. Hodsman AB, Kiessel M, Watson PH, et al. Bone histomorphometric changes after 2 years of cyclic parathyroid hormone treatment in women with osteoporosis [abstract]. Bone 1998; 23: S631
75. Cosman F, Nieves J, Woelfert L, et al. Alendronate does not block the anabolic effect of PTH in postmenopausal osteoporotic women. J Bone Miner Res 1998; 13: 1051-5
76. Hodsman AB, Drost D, Fraher LJ, et al. The addition of a raloxifene analog (LY117018) allows for reduced PTH(1-34) dosing during reversal of osteopenia in ovariectomized rats. J Bone Miner Res 1999; 14: 675-9
77. Hodsman AB, Watson PH, Drost D, et al. Assessment of maintenance therapy with reduced doses of PTH-(1-34) in combination with a raloxifene analogue (LY117018) following anabolic therapy in the ovariectomized rat. Bone 1999; 24: 451-5
78. Rittmaster RS, Bolognese M, Ettinger M, et al. Treatment of osteoporosis with parathyroid hormone followed by alendronate: bone density results [abstract]. Bone 1998; 23: S517
79. Delman PD, Vergnaud P, Arlot ME, et al. The anabolic effect of human PTH-(1-34) on bone formation is blunted when bone resorption is inhibited by the bisphosphonate tiludronate: is activated resorption a prerequisite for the in vivo effect of PTH on formation in a remodelling system? Bone 1995; 16: 603-10
80. Whitfield JF, Morley P, Willick GE, et al. Stimulation of femoral trabecular bone growth by human parathyroid hormone (hPTH)-(1-30)NH_2. Calcif Tissue Int. In press
81. Mohan S, Kutilek S, Zhang C, et al. Evidence that PTH effects on bone formation may involve modulation of PKA pathway while its effects on bone resorption may involve modulation of PKC pathway in a mouse model [abstract]. Bone 1998; 23: S449
82. Fraher LJ, Avram R, Watson PH, et al. A comparison of the biochemical responses to 1-31 hPTH and –34 hPTH given to healthy humans by slow infusion. J Clin Endocrinol Metab. In press
83. Whitfield JF. Calcium: cell cycle driver, differentiator and killer. Austin (TX): Landes Bioscience, 1997
84. Werner H, LeRoith D. The insulin-like growth factor receptor signaling pathways are important for tumorigenesis and inhibition of apoptosis. Crit Rev Oncog 1997; 8: 71-92

Correspondence: Dr *James F. Whitfield*, Institute for Biological Sciences, National Research Council of Canada, Building M-54, Montréal Road Campus, Ottawa, Ontario K1A 0R6, Canada.
E-mail: pthosteo@home.com

Efficacy and Tolerability of Calcitonin in the Prevention and Treatment of Osteoporosis

Véronique Halkin[1] and *Jean-Yves Reginster*[1,2]

1 Bone and Cartilage Metabolism Unit, University of Liège, Liège, Belgium
2 Georgetown University Medical Center, Washington, DC, USA

1. Pharmacological Properties

Since its discovery more than 30 years ago, calcitonin has been extensively tested both in animals and humans. In humans, calcitonin is mainly produced by the C cells of the thyroid[1] and is a polypeptide containing 32 amino acid residues.

1.1 Relative Activity

There are several differences in the amino acid composition of the calcitonins from different species, and these are associated with different potencies.[2] The biological activity of different calcitonins is expressed in MRC (Medical Research Council) units, also called IU (International Units).[3] It is measured through induction of hypocalcaemia at 1 hour after injection in a standardised model using young rats. The mass corresponding to 1 unit of calcitonin differs widely from species to species. Eel and salmon calcitonins have the highest activity/weight ratio. Pig and human calcitonins have a weaker effect for the same weight. An assessment of the relative potencies of various calcitonins reveals that calcitonins from teleostean fish are 50 to 100 times more potent than those from mammals, and also have a longer duration of hypocalcaemic activity.

1.2 Endogenous Calcitonin

Secretion of endogenous calcitonin is modulated by many factors. These include blood calcium level, which is the main physiological factor regulating calcitonin secretion. Calcitonin inhibits bone resorption and thereby lowers plasma calcium. Calcitonin is a calcium-regulating hormone with a negative feedback mechanism. Calcitonin also seems to belong to the neuro-endocrine system. Receptors to calcitonin have been found in the central nervous system.

1.3 Exogenous Calcitonin

Because of its anti-osteoclastic and analgesic properties, calcitonin is a first line choice in the treatment of several bone diseases characterised by absolute or relative bone resorption.

1.3.1 Effects on Bone

All calcitonins have an anti-osteoclastic property. Osteoclasts possess specific receptors that bind calcitonin. Administration of calcitonin causes the brush border of the osteoclasts to disappear and the osteoclasts to move away from the bone resorption surface. Calcitonin radically alters the internal structure of isolated osteoclasts, inhibiting cytoplasmic mobility, which is essential for bone resorption. Finally, calcitonin reduces the lifespan and number of osteoclasts, probably by decreasing their rate of formation by blocking the fusion of mononuclear marrow cells, the committed progenitors of the osteoclasts that are known to possess calcitonin receptors.

Zimolo et al.[4] demonstrated a quantifiable pharmacological effect of calcitonin on single osteoclasts. They were able to show in animal models that Na^+-independent acid extrusion is stimulated by osteoclast attachment to bone and is virtually absent when osteoclasts are treated with salcatonin.

1.3.2 Routes of Delivery

For many years, it was necessary to administer calcitonin parenterally, by either intramuscular or subcutaneous injection. With respect to the prevention and treatment of postmenopausal osteoporosis, the chronic nature of the disease and the subsequent long duration of the pharmacological intervention required uncomfortable repetitive long term administration. New routes of administration have therefore been developed. Rectal administration is very efficient, but does not seem to be well accepted from a social or personal standpoint. Oral administration of polypeptide hormones is precluded because of gastrointestinal digestion; at present, the most promising delivery method is that of nasal spray. In a recent review,[5] it was concluded from comparative studies evaluating the effects of intranasal and parenteral salcatonin in healthy volunteers that equivalent biochemical effects are obtained when the intranasal dosage is approximately 2 to 4 times that of the parenteral dosage, although full dose-response curves are not concurrently available for the 2 routes of administration.

2. Therapeutic Efficacy

2.1 Prevention of Osteoporosis

Currently, salcatonin is being explored and used in the prevention and treatment of postmenopausal osteoporosis and in acute post-ovariectomy osteoporosis. Calcitonin was also shown to be effective in senile, immobilisation-induced and corticosteroid-induced forms of osteoporosis.[6] In most randomised studies in which intranasal salcatonin (usually 50 to 200 IU/day) plus oral calcium supplements were administered for 1 to 5 years to recently postmenopausal women for prevention of osteoporosis, bone mineral density or content of the lumbar spine increased by approximately 1 to 3% from baseline, compared with a reduction of approximately 3 to 6% among women receiving oral calcium supplements only.[5] A long term evaluation of a low-dose intermittent intranasal salcatonin regimen (50 IU/day for 5 days/week) demonstrated a statistically significant difference in favour of salcatonin plus calcium over calcium alone in bone mineral density of lumbar vertebrae after 6 months; this was maintained for the entire duration of the 5-year study.[7] Concerning the effect of nasal calcitonin on cortical bone, the conclusions are variable, ranging from a protective effect of calcitonin 100 IU/day without calcium supplementation[8] to an absence of efficacy in similar conditions[9] or with high doses of up to 400 IU/day with calcium supplements.[10]

One double-blind study of whether intranasal salcatonin prevents physiological bone loss at perimenopause concluded that nasal salcatonin 100 IU/day had no protective effect on bone mass and does not modify bone metabolism at perimenopause.[11]

To observe a significant reduction of fracture rate, osteoporosis prevention therapy needs to be administered for at least 5 to 10 years,[12] with the implication that if a drug is given in an injectable form a higher dropout rate is observed. This was the case when human calcitonin was given to healthy postmenopausal women who had to perform subcutaneous auto-injections.[13]

Two studies employing animal models were used to evaluate the effect of calcitonin on bone quality *in vivo*. In adult ewes, intermittent calcitonin treatment from the time of ovariectomy was associated with a significant preservation of cancellous bone strength and strain in trabecular bone of the femoral neck, without affecting the crystalline properties of bone.[14] Similarly, the administration of salcatonin to rabbits improves the biochemical properties of normal bone and after osteotomy.[15]

Most studies in recently postmenopausal healthy women show that intranasal calcitonin plus oral calcium produce mild to moderate reductions in biochemical markers of bone turnover.[5,16] However, some trials showed nonsignificant changes in biochemical markers of bone turnover despite attenuation of reduction in bone mineral density or content with salcatonin.[7,11,17,18]

The efficacy of calcitonin in the prevention of secondary (glucocorticoid-induced) osteoporosis has been studied. Prevention in patients commencing corticosteroids has been investigated by different authors.[19-21] The double-blind placebo-controlled study by Adachi et al.[19] concluded that calcitonin nasal spray 200 IU/day prevented early bone loss in the lumbar spine in half of the corticosteroid-treated patients. However, Sambrook et al.[20] did not show any additional benefit of adding calcitonin to calcitriol or cholecalciferol in the prevention of glucocorticoid-induced osteoporosis.

2.2 Treatment of Established Osteoporosis

Several authors have demonstrated a positive effect of calcitonin on established osteoporosis. The efficacy of the injectable form of calcitonin has been confirmed in the treatment of postmenopausal osteoporosis in short term uncontrolled studies,[22,23] as well as in long term studies.[24] In an open prospective study, Rico et al.[25] suggested that the administration of intramuscular salcatonin 100 IU/day, plus 500mg of elemental calcium, for 10 days each month significantly reduced the number of new vertebral fractures compared with those women receiving only calcium. A significant increase in trabecular bone and cortical bone was also observed in this trial. The authors suggested that salcatonin is effective in the treatment of osteoporosis with a specific action on both cortical and trabecular bone.[25]

Overgaard et al.[26] evaluated the outcome of salcatonin nasal spray therapy in a well designed 2-year parallel-group trial in terms of the proportion of patients who responded in each treatment group. The subanalysis demonstrated that the benefits of salcatonin nasal spray therapy were seen in the majority of women, and that salcatonin nasal spray represents an effective therapeutic alternative for osteoporotic women who are postmenopausal for more than 5 years, who decline or do not tolerate estrogens, or for whom estrogens are contraindicated. The randomised double-blind placebo-controlled trial by Ellerington et al.[17] reached the same conclusion. The positive results obtained with calcitonin in the treatment of postmenopausal osteoporosis also seem to apply to glucocorticoid-induced osteoporosis, as shown by Ringe et al.[27] in a randomised open study.

The large PROOF study[28] confirms the above conclusion. In this 5-year, multicentre, double-blind randomised study involving 1175 women with established osteoporosis, an interim analysis after 3 years showed a significant reduction in the relative risk of new vertebral fractures for women treated with nasal salcatonin 200 IU/day, while the level of statistical significance was not reached for lower or higher dosages.

2.3 Calcitonin Escape Phenomenon and Calcitonin Antibodies

Long term administration of salcatonin can lead to resistance to the hormone and subsequent reduction of efficacy.[5] The amino acid sequence of salcatonin differs considerably from that of the human hormone, and specific antibodies develop in a significant proportion of patients after parenteral or nasal administration of nasal salcatonin. Controversy remains regarding the functional importance of these antibodies. We investigated the development of specific anti-salcatonin antibodies in a population of postmenopausal women receiving salcatonin for prevention of postmenopausal bone loss.[29] The effect of salcatonin in women with or without antibodies were compared. No significant differences were discovered between the two groups. We concluded that antibodies do not alter the efficacy of salcatonin on bone. Takahashi et al.[30] suggested another mechanism to explain the reduction of efficacy, including a downregulation of the skeletal receptor for calcitonin, which may provide a more plausible explanation for the so-called 'calcitonin-escape' phenomenon.

3. Tolerability and Safety

For many years, it has been necessary to administer calcitonin parenterally by either intramuscular or subcutaneous injections. Unfortunately, there are several drawbacks to injections. In some cases, the injection of calcitonin produces unpleasant reactions. The most frequent adverse effect is nausea, which occurs shortly after injection in up to 30% of patients. This phenomenon may last for several hours or even until the next injection. Evening administration with concomitant antiemetics can bring relief to some extent. Other symptoms include local pain at the site of injection, flushing, diarrhoea and vomiting, and are the cause for stopping long term treatment in approximately 45% of patients.

In contrast, administration by nasal spray is often well tolerated, and none of the adverse effects experienced during parenteral administration of the hormone are observed even in patients who had discontinued the drug when it was previously administered by injection.[31] Nasal spray does not cause pathological abnormalities at the site of administration.[32] Calcitonin appears to be very well tolerated, and no evidence of systemic toxicity has been observed to date.

4. Dosage and Administration

The frequency and amount of calcitonin to administer in prevention as well as in treatment of osteoporosis is still under investigation. It seems that in established osteoporosis there is a dose-dependent effect on the trabecular[33,34] and cortical bone mass.[33] The nasal bioavailability of salcatonin is only 10 to 25% in comparison with subcutaneous or intramuscular injection, but the biological effects of the nasal spray of calcitonin represent 40% of those observed with the injectable form.[35-38]

In prevention of osteoporosis, there is some nonconclusive evidence relating to the minimal effective dosage of salcatonin needed to prevent bone loss. We performed a double-blind placebo-controlled randomised study of 3 parallel groups who received intranasal salcatonin 50 or 200IU, or placebo, on 5 days/week.[18] Salcatonin 50 IU/day prevented lumbar bone loss, and 200 IU/day resulted in a significant increase in lumbar bone mineral density. In the treatment of established osteoporosis, Rico et al.[25] suggested that intramuscular salcatonin 100 IU/day plus 500mg of elemental calcium for 10 days each month is effective, with a specific action on both cortical and trabecular bone.

Long term administration of intranasal salcatonin can increase bone mass at the lumbar spine at the rate of 1% for each 100 IU of calcitonin per day after 2 years.[33] The PROOF study suggests that the combination of 200IU of salcatonin, 1000mg of calcium and 400IU of vitamin D is able to reduce significantly the relative risk of new vertebral fractures compared with placebo.[28]

5. Calcitonin in the Management of Pain

In addition to its positive effect on bone mass, calcitonin has a significant analgesic effect generally. However, there is no consensus concerning the mechanism of action involved in the analgesic effect, which has been shown with human, salmon and eel calcitonins.[39-42] Nasal salcatonin 200 IU/day in established osteoporosis possesses a potent analgesic effect, reduces the duration of bed confinement and decreases the number of concomitant analgesic medications.[35,37]

References

1. Wolffe HJ. Calcitonin; perspective in current concepts. J Endocrinol Invest 1982; 5: 523-30
2. MacIntyre I, Craig R. Molecular evolution of the calcitonins. In: Fink G, Whalley, J, editors. Neuropeptides: basic and clinical aspects. London: Churchill Livingstone, 1982: 255-8
3. Gaines Das RE, Zanelli JM. The international reference preparation of calcitonin, human, for bioassay: assessment of material and definition of the international unit. Acta Endocrinol 1980; 93: 37-42
4. Zimolo Z, Wesolowski G, Rodan AG. Acid extrusion is induced by osteoclast attachment to bone. J Clin Invest 1995; 96: 2277-83
5. Plosker GL, McTavish D. Intranasal salcatonin: a review of its pharmacological properties and in the management of postmenopausal osteoporosis. Drugs Aging 1996; 8: 378-400
6. Reginster JY. Ostéoporose postménopausique: traitement prophylactique. Paris: Masson, 1993; 127-37
7. Reginster JY, Meurmans L, Deroisy R, et al. A 5-year controlled randomized study of prevention of postmenopausal trabecular bone loss with nasal salmon calcitonin and calcium. Eur J Clin Invest 1994; 24: 565-9
8. Ribot C, Tremollieres F, Pouilles JM, et al. Long-term effect of nasal calcitonin on vertebral and femoral bone mass in early menopause : results of a controlled prospective 3-year study. J Bone Miner Res 1992; 7 Suppl. 1: 196
9. Gennari C, Chierichetti SM, Bigazzi S, et al. Comparative effects on bone mineral content of calcium and calcium plus calcitonin given into different regimens in postmenopausal osteoporosis. Curr Ther Res 1985; 38: 455-64
10. Overgaard K, Hansen MA, Christiansen C. Effect of intranasal calcitonin on bone mass and bone turnover in early postmenopausal women: a dose-response study. J Bone Miner Res 1992; 7 Suppl. 1: 140
11. Arnala I, Saastamoinen J, Alhava EM. Salmon calcitonin in the prevention of bone loss at perimenopause. Bone 1996; 4 Suppl. 6: 629-632
12. Christiansen C, Lindsay R. Estrogens, bone loss and preservation. Osteoporos Int 1991; 1: 7-14
13. McIntyre I, Stevenson JC, Whitehead MI, et al. Calcitonin for prevention of postmenopausal bone loss. Lancet 1988; I: 900-2
14. Geusens P, Boonen S, Nijs J. Effect of salmon calcitonin on femoral bone quality in adult ovariectomized ewes. Calcif Tissue Int 1996; 59: 315-20
15. Karachalios T, Lyritis GP, Giannarakos DG. Calcitonin effects on rabbit bone. Acta Orthop Scand 1992; 63: 615-8
16. Lyritis G, Magiasis B, Tsakalakos N. Prevention of bone loss in early nonsurgical and nonosteoporotic high turnover patients with salmon calcitonin: the role of biochemical bone markers in monitoring high turnover patients under calcitonin treatment. Calcif Tissue Int 1995; 56: 38-41

17. Ellerington MC, Hillard TC, Whitcroft SIJ. Intranasal salmon calcitonin for the prevention and treatment of postmenopausal osteoporosis. Calcif Tissue Int 1996; 59: 6-11
18. Reginster JY, Deroisy R, Lecart MP, et al. A double-blind, placebo-controlled, dose-finding trial of intermittent nasal salmon calcitonin for prevention of postmenopausal lumbar spine bone loss. Am J Med 1995; 98: 452-8
19. Adachi JD, Bensen WG, Bell MJ, et al. Salmon calcitonin nasal spray in the prevention of corticosteroid-induced osteoporosis. Br J Rheumatol 1997; 36: 255-9
20. Sambrook P, Birmingham J, Kelly P, et al. Prevention of corticosteroid osteoporosis: comparison of calcium, calcitriol and calcitonin. N Engl J Med 1993; 328: 1747-52
21. Kotaniemi A, Piirainen H, Paimela L, et al. Intranasal salmon calcitonin (sCT) prevents bone loss in active rheumatoid arthritis (RA) with low dose glucocorticoids [abstract]. Arthritis Rheum 1994; 37 Suppl. 9: 288
22. Canniggia A, Gennari C, Bencini M, et al. Calcium metabolism and 47-calcium kinetics before and after long-term thyrocalcitonin treatment in senile osteoporosis. Clin Sci 1970; 38: 397-407
23. Milhaud G, Talbot JN, Coutris G. Calcitonin treatment of postmenopausal osteoporosis, evaluation of efficacy by principal component analysis. Biomedicine 1975; 23: 223-32
24. Reginster JY. Calcitonin for prevention and treatment of osteoporosis. Am J Med 1993; 95 Suppl. 1: 44-7
25. Rico H, Revilla M, Hernandez ER, et al. Total and regional bone mineral content and fracture rate in postmenopausal osteoporosis treated with salmon calcitonin: a prospective study. Calcif Tissue Int 1995; 56: 181-5
26. Overgaard K, Lindsay R, Christiansen C. Patient responsiveness to calcitonin salmon nasal spray: a subanalysis of a 2-year study. Clin Ther 1995; 17: 680-5
27. Ringe JD, Welzel D. Salmon calcitonin in the therapy of corticoid-induced osteoporosis. Eur J Clin Pharmacol 1987; 33: 35-9
28. Stock JL, Avioli LV, Baylink DJ. Calcitonin-salmon nasal spray reduces the incidence of new vertebral fractures in postmenopausal women: three-year interim results of the PROOF study [abstract no. 187]. J Bone Miner Res 1997; 12 Suppl. 1: S149
29. Reginster JY, Gaspard S, Deroisy R. Prevention of osteoporosis with nasal salmon calcitonin: effect of anti-salmon calcitonin antibody formation. Osteoporos Int 1993; 3: 261-4
30. Takahashi S, Goldring S, Katz M, et al. Down-regulation of calcitonin receptor mRNA expression by calcitonin during human osteoclast-like cell differentiation. J Clin Invest 1995; 95: 167-71
31. Reginster JY, Franchimont P. Side-effects of synthetic salmon calcitonin given by intranasal spray compared with intramuscular injection. Clin Exp Rheumatol 1985; 3: 155-7
32. Foti R, Martorana U, Broggini M. Long-term tolerability of nasal spray formulation of salmon calcitonin. Curr Ther Res 1995; 56 Suppl. 4: 429-35
33. Overgaard K, Hansen MA, Jensen SB, et al. Effect of salcatonin given intranasally on bone mass and fracture rates in established osteoporosis: a dose-response study. BMJ 1992; 305: 556-61
34. Thamsborg G, Storm TL, Sykulski R, et al. Effect of different doses of nasal salmon calcitonin on bone mass. Calcif Tissue Int 1991; 41: 302-7
35. Nagant De Deuxchaisnes C, Devogelaer JP, Huaux JP, et al. New modes of administration of salmon calcitonin in Paget's disease. Clin Orthop Relat Res 1987; 217: 56-71
36. Overgaard K, Agnusdei D, Hansen MA, et al. Dose-response bioactivity of salmon calcitonin in premenopausal and postmenopausal women. J Clin Endocrinol Metab 1991; 72: 344-9
37. Reginster JY, Denis D, Albert A, et al. Assessment of the biological effectiveness of nasal synthetic salmon calcitonin (SSCT) by comparison with intramuscular (im) or placebo injection in normal subjects. Bone Miner 1987; 2: 133-40
38. Mazzuoli GF, Passeri M, Gennari C, et al. Effects of salmon calcitonin in postmenopausal osteoporosis; a controlled double-blind study. Calcif Tissue Int 1986; 38: 3-8
39. Guidobono F, Netti C, Villani P, et al. Antinociceptive activity of eel calcitonin, injected into the inflamed paw in rats. Neuropharmacology 1991; 30; 1275-8
40. Ljunghall S, Gardsell P, Johnell O, et al. Synthetic human calcitonin in postmenopausal osteoporosis: a placebo-controlled, double-blind study. Calcif Tissue Int 1991; 49: 17-9
41. Lyritis GP, Tsakalakos N, Magiasis B, et al. Analgesic effect of salmon calcitonin in osteoporotic vertebral fractures: a double blind placebo-controlled clinical study. Calcif Tissue Int 1991; 49: 369-72
42. Pun KK, Shan LWL. Analgesic effect of salmon calcitonin in the treatment of osteoporotic vertebral fractures. Clin Ther 1989; 11: 205-9

Correspondence: Dr *Jean-Yves Reginster*, Bone and Cartilage Metabolism Unit, Policliniques L Brull, CHU Centre-Ville, Quai Godefroid Kurth 45 (+9), 4020 Liège, Belgium.

Selective Estrogen Receptor Modulators
A Look Ahead

Bruce H. Mitlak[1,2] and *Fredric J. Cohen*[2]

1 Indiana University School of Medicine, Indianapolis, Indiana, USA
2 Eli Lilly and Company, Indianapolis, Indiana, USA

The search for more acceptable and safer alternatives to postmenopausal hormone replacement therapies has led to the evaluation of compounds known as selective estrogen receptor modulators (SERMs). SERMs are a group of structurally diverse compounds that bind to estrogen receptors (ER) and elicit responses which are either similar to or distinct from those seen when 17β-estradiol (the prototypical estrogen) is bound to ER, depending on the specific cellular and hormonal milieu.[1] While SERMS work through ER, other drugs with estrogen antagonist effects do not work directly via the ER, including aromatase inhibitors and gonadotropin-releasing hormone (GnRH) agonists.[1a] In contrast to SERMS, which have selective agonist or antagonist activity, so-called 'pure antiestrogens', such as the steroidal compound ICI 182,780 (Faslodex®), binds to ER but elicits a largely ER antagonist profile in estrogen-response tissues.

Based on accumulating clinical trial evidence, several SERMs are being evaluated for the prevention and/or treatment of hormone-responsive cancer, for prevention and/or treatment of postmenopausal osteoporosis and for prevention and/or treatment of cardiovascular disease and other estrogen deficiency–related indications. Given the multiple potential target tissues of SERMs (i.e. all that contain ER), it is important to define the actions of each SERM individually, not only with respect to genitourinary and reproductive tissues but also with regard to effects on the skeletal, cardiovascular and nervous systems. In anticipation of new SERMs and related compounds to treat or prevent diseases important for postmenopausal women, new guidelines for their clinical evaluation are being formulated by various regulatory and public health organisations.[2]

The evolving clinical data on several SERMs have been paralleled by remarkable advances in the understanding of the mechanisms of action for these compounds. For example, work in the field of ER biology, including solution of the crystalline structure of the ERα ligand-binding domain,[3] provides insight into the molecular basis of SERM specificity and is consistent with extensive structure-activity studies on these compounds.[4-6] This chapter briefly reviews the molecular basis of SERM activity, highlighting recent molecular biological findings and future areas of research, presents available clinical data on these compounds and concludes with a glimpse towards the more distant future.

1. Molecular Basis For Tissue-Specific Actions Via the Estrogen Receptor

Estrogen receptors (ER) were first identified[7] and isolated[8] in the 1960s. They are ligand-inducible nuclear transcription factors, which are physiologically activated by steroids (e.g. estradiol, estrone, etc.) but which can also be activated by a large variety of nonsteroidal ligands.[9] Two unique ER isoforms (ERα and ERβ) have been cloned in humans and rodents, and the structural domains for both have been described.[10] Additionally, many naturally occurring ER variants and mutants, especially those found in human breast cancer, have been described.[11]

At least two regions of ER are required for transcriptional activity: activating function-1 (AF-1), located near the amino terminus; and activating function-2 (AF-2), located within the ligand-binding domain.[12,13] A third putative independent activating function (AF-2a), also located within the ligand-binding region, was recently described.[14] One or more of these activating functions may be required for SERM gene transactivation, depending on the cell and gene promoter context.[12,15] Importantly, the ability to affect differentially the three-dimensional structure of the AF-2 region after ligand binding has been proposed as an important mechanism contributing to the selective actions of different ER ligands.[3,16,17]

A solution to the crystalline structure of the ligand-binding domain of ERα (after binding to either 17β-estradiol or to raloxifene) has been reported.[3] A key feature of the structure is the ability of ERα helix 12 in the ligand-binding site (an essential site for AF-2 activation) to fold into the complex after estradiol is bound. This presumably allows AF-2 to activate gene transcription at the estrogen response element (ERE) upon estradiol-ER binding. Despite similar coordination of raloxifene in the ER ligand-binding pocket, the raloxifene alkyl aminoethoxy side chain displaces helix 12 via direct interaction with aspartate 351 of ERα, presumably rendering AF-2 incapable of activating ERE-driven gene transcription. This observation physically accounts for the well known ability of ER antagonists, such as raloxifene, to block E_2 activation of ERE-driven genes by blocking AF-2 activity.[16] In support of this hypothesis, Levenson and Jordan[18] have shown that a naturally occurring ER mutant derived from human breast cancer cells (in which aspartate 351 is replaced by tyrosine), when transfected into ER-negative breast cancer cells, changes raloxifene from an ER antagonist into an ER agonist, at least with respect to gene activation of transforming growth factor-α.

The nature of the ER ligand is clearly not the only factor that accounts for SERM tissue specificity. Current areas of research are concentrated on several other crucial factors, including: gene-specific pathways for ER-mediated gene transcription which do not depend upon a consensus ERE,[19-21] the cell-selective presence of ERβ, a recently described isoform of the ER,[10,22,23] and the cell- and/or gene-specific presence of activating or inhibiting protein cofactors and chromatin remodelling proteins (i.e. coactivators and corepressors), which regulate ER-mediated gene transcription.[5,24,25]

2. Selective Estrogen Receptor Modulators (SERMs) Currently Approved or in Clinical Development

A number of synthetic compounds display mixed ER agonist/antagonist profiles and thereby provide potential estrogen-like specificity to the skeleton and cardiovascular system. Nonsteroidal SERMs now in development include triphenylethylene, benzothiophene, naphthalene, chroman, indole and benzopyran compounds, among others (fig. 1).

2.1 Tamoxifen

Tamoxifen, a triphenylethylene, was synthesised and developed in the 1960s,[26,27] and first reports of its use for the treatment of advanced breast cancer appeared in the early 1970s.[28]

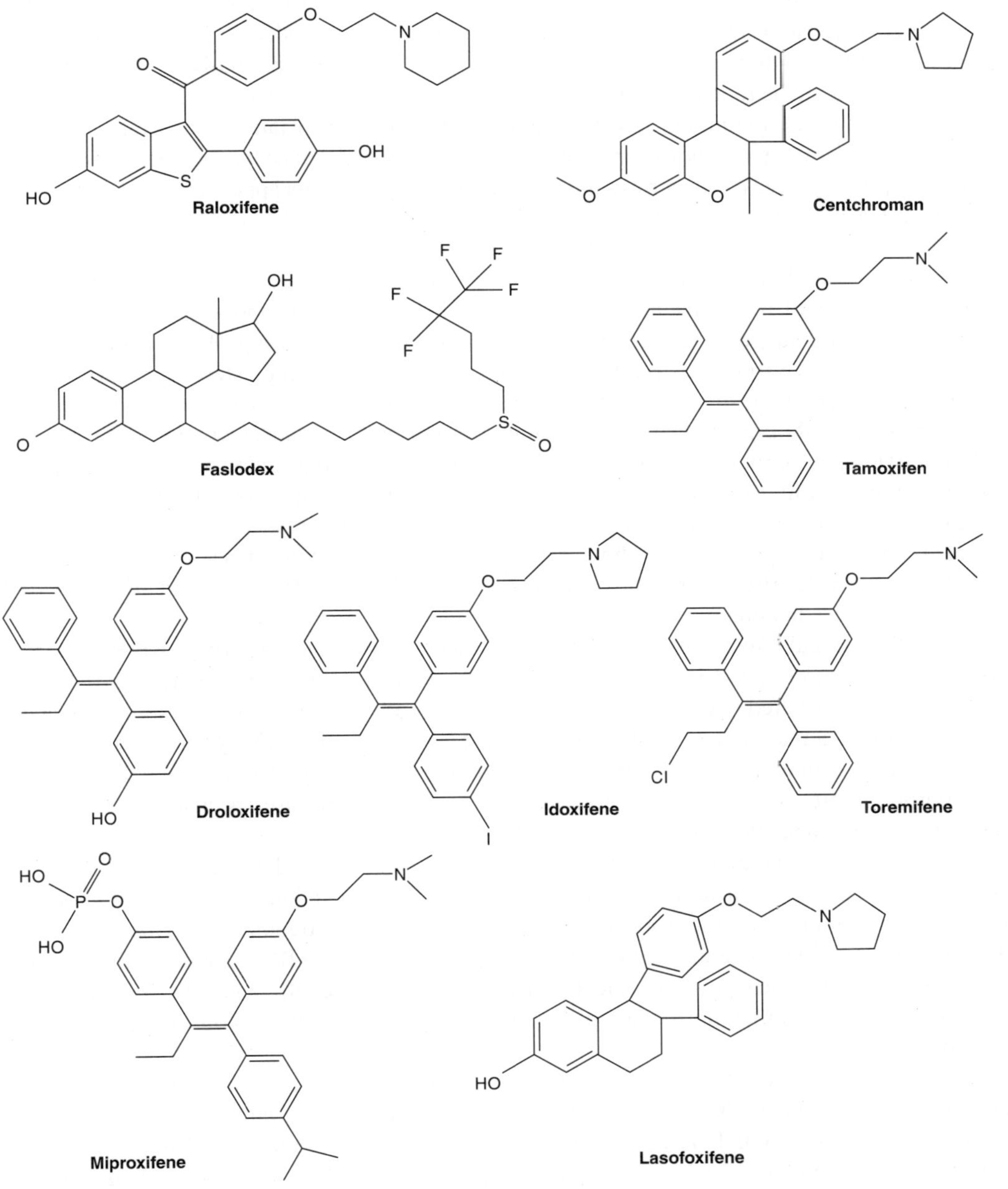

Raloxifene

Centchroman

Faslodex

Tamoxifen

Droloxifene

Idoxifene

Toremifene

Miproxifene

Lasofoxifene

Fig. 1. Chemical structure of selected selective estrogen receptor modulators and the pure antiestrogen Faslodex®.

Currently, tamoxifen is the endocrine treatment of choice for advanced breast cancer as well as for adjuvant therapy to surgery, radiation and chemotherapy in earlier disease stages, with an estimated 8 to 10 million patient-years of experience for this use. In the adjuvant therapy of breast cancer, use of tamoxifen for at least 5 years is recommended, since this affords the greatest reductions in disease-free (≈45%) and overall (≈25%) survival relative to no adjuvant therapy.[29] Data on the long term follow-up of women with breast cancer receiving tamoxifen for more than 5 years are limited, and the optimal duration of adjuvant tamoxifen therapy remains controversial.[29] Importantly, however, the benefit of tamoxifen to reduce the incidence of contralateral (i.e. primary) breast cancer by as much as 40% in these patients appears to be maintained through at least 10 years of continuous use.[30]

In addition to its ER antagonist properties in breast malignancy, tamoxifen has ER agonist properties in the skeleton, uterus and cardiovascular system. For example, tamoxifen preserves spine and hip bone mineral density (BMD) in postmenopausal breast cancer patients,[31,32] and may also reduce their risk of coronary heart disease (CHD).[33] Tamoxifen has also been shown to preserve BMD[34,35] and to lower serum cholesterol [primarily low density lipoprotein-cholesterol (LDL-C)][36] in studies of healthy postmenopausal women. As opposed to the BMD-preserving effects of tamoxifen in postmenopausal women, two trials in reproductive-aged women have shown decreases in BMD during tamoxifen therapy at the radius, spine and hip.[35,37] Tamoxifen thus appears to have estrogen-like effects on bone in the presence of low circulating estrogen levels, but ER antagonist effects when circulating estrogen levels are high. These findings suggest that the prevailing estrogen milieu directly affects the ultimate effects of tamoxifen in bone, implicating ER as a direct mediator of tamoxifen activity in bone.

The US National Cancer Institute's Breast Cancer Prevention Trial (NSABP P-1 trial), which enrolled more that 13 000 otherwise healthy women who were at increased risk for breast cancer, was halted after a mean follow-up of 48 months. Results from this study indicate that tamoxifen decreases the risk of invasive breast cancer by about 45% overall (the benefit confined to a reduction in risk of ER-positive tumours) and may also decrease the risk of osteoporotic fractures.[38] There was no effect of tamoxifen on disease-specific mortality, but the trial was not adequately sized to detect such an effect.

Two other trials (one in the UK, one in Italy), each much smaller than NSABP P-1, did not find a significant effect of tamoxifen on breast cancer risk reduction.[39,40] There are at least three reasons accounting for these apparently discrepant results: the populations in the European prevention trials were different from each other and from the NSABP P-1 cohort; the Italian trial had limited statistical power to detect even a robust clinical benefit; and both trials allowed women to use concomitant hormone replacement therapy (HRT), perhaps obscuring a benefit of tamoxifen.

Unfortunately, there are several limitations to the long term use of tamoxifen in healthy, postmenopausal women. In women with or without breast cancer, tamoxifen significantly increases the risk of vaginal discharge and endometrial cancer incidence by as much as 6-fold over placebo after prolonged use.[30,38] Tamoxifen also significantly increases the risk of venous thromboembolism (deep vein thrombosis and pulmonary embolism), to a degree similar to that of during estrogen replacement therapy (ERT).[30,38] It also causes vasomotor symptoms (i.e. hot flashes) which can be severe enough to lead to discontinuation of therapy in a minority of breast cancer patients.[41,42] The severity of tamoxifen-related hot flashes was determined in healthy women (both pre- and postmenopausal) in the P-1 trial via directed questionnaire. 46% of all women receiving tamoxifen reported having at least one hot flash episode that was 'quite a bit bothersome' (a rating of 3 on a 4-point scale) or worse severity compared with 29% of women receiving placebo.[38]

2.2 Toremifene

Toremifene is approved for the treatment of advanced breast cancer in postmenopausal women in several countries including the US. It has been directly compared to tamoxifen in prospective clinical trials of previously untreated postmenopausal breast cancer patients (ER-positive or ER-unknown) and has been shown to have similar efficacy and adverse effects.[43] The ER agonist properties of toremifene have been less thoroughly studied. In a randomised trial comparing toremifene with tamoxifen in 49 postmenopausal women with node-positive breast cancer, both compounds lowered serum total and LDL-C and lipoprotein (a).[44] In contrast to tamoxifen, toremifene increased high density lipoprotein-cholesterol (HDL-C) by 14%. In another report from Finland, toremifene 40 mg/day was shown to have a similar but weaker effect on biochemical markers of bone metabolism and BMD than tamoxifen 20 mg/day in 30 postmenopausal women with breast cancer. In the latter report, a marker of bone degradation, urinary cross-linked amino terminal telopeptide of type I collagen (NTx) was decreased by 33% and 16% in the patients receiving tamoxifen and toremifene after 1 year, respectively, while osteocalcin, a marker of overall bone turnover was suppressed 25% by tamoxifen but not by toremifene.[45] In the same patients, BMD increased by an average of 1% at the hip and 2% at the lumbar spine after 1 year in the patients receiving tamoxifen but did not increase in the patients receiving toremifene.

2.3 Other Tamoxifen Derivatives

Three other triphenylethylene derivatives, droloxifene (3-hydroxytamoxifen), idoxifene (pyrollidino-4-iodotamoxifen) and miproxifene (TAT-59) have also been evaluated clinically (fig. 1). A phase II study demonstrated the antitumour activity of droloxifene in postmenopausal women with advanced breast cancer.[46] The clinical development of droloxifene for breast cancer and other uses in postmenopausal women was completely halted in 1999, after the drug had advanced to phase III. The reasons given for stopping included insufficient efficacy to treat breast cancer and a relatively unfavourable profile compared with lasofoxifene (see below).[47] Idoxifene was in phase III testing for osteoporosis prevention and in phase II testing for breast cancer treatment when its development was halted.[47a] Clinical data at the time development was halted indicated a profile similar to that of tamoxifen.[48-50] Miproxifene is in phase III trials in Japan for treatment of advanced breast cancer. The effects of miproxifene on the skeleton, cardiovascular system and the uterus in postmenopausal women have not been reported.

2.4 Levormeloxifene

Levormeloxifene is the *l*-enantiomer of racemic centchroman (fig. 1).[51] Centchroman has been used for about the past 20 years as a postcoital contraceptive, particularly in India, where it was originally developed. The *l*-enantiomer has a 7-fold higher binding affinity for ER as compared with the *d*-enantiomer and also has an approximately 7-fold higher uterotrophic activity in sexually immature rats not treated with estrogen.[52] When such rats are first treated with subcutaneous E_2, levormeloxifene maximally inhibited the uterotrophic activity of E_2 by only 40%. Thus, under these conditions, levormeloxifene is a partial agonist of ER in the rat uterus.[52]

There are limited clinical data on levormeloxifene, none published in a peer-reviewed journal. Clinical development of levormeloxifene was terminated during phase III testing for prevention and treatment of postmenopausal osteoporosis, reportedly because of concerns over uterine stimulation and an increase in uterovaginal prolapse with urinary incontinence.[58]

2.5 Benzothiophenes

Raloxifene binds with high affinity to both ERα and ERβ.[59,60] Clinical trials indicate that raloxifene has ER agonist effects on bone and serum lipids in healthy, postmenopausal women, and it has been approved for osteoporosis prevention and treatment in several countries. Raloxifene 60 mg/day after 4 and 31 weeks reduced urinary calcium excretion and bone resorption and produced improvements in total body calcium balance[61] in early postmenopausal women, similar to the effects observed in women treated with cyclic HRT (0.625 mg/day conjugated equine estrogens, 5 mg/day medroxyprogesterone).

In a multicentre, randomised and double-blind trial, raloxifene 60 mg/day for 24 months significantly increased BMD from baseline values. Differences in BMD between the raloxifene and placebo groups were 2.4% in the lumbar spine and total hip and 2.0% in the total body. Associated with these changes in BMD, serum levels of bone-specific alkaline phosphatase and osteocalcin decreased by 23.1 and 15.0%, respectively, and urinary type I collagen C-telopeptide/creatinine excretion decreased by 34%.

Hot flashes were characterised in an analysis of three raloxifene trials (n = 876 healthy postmenopausal women, mean age of 54 years). After 30 months of follow-up, the cumulative incidence of hot flashes was 21% for placebo and 28% for raloxifene (p = 0.022), and the difference in incidence rate was limited to the first 6 months of therapy. There was no therapy difference for maximum severity or total duration of hot flashes, or early discontinuation due to hot flashes.[62] In an analysis of 1145 healthy postmenopausal women, 3 years of raloxifene therapy (at doses ranging from 30 to 150 mg/day) did not increase vaginal bleeding, spotting or other uterine-related adverse events, and did not increase endometrial thickness or the incidence of uterine pathology compared with placebo.[62a] In a 1-year study comparing raloxifene 60 or 150 mg/day with placebo and conjugated estrogens 0.625 mg/day, raloxifene did not stimulate the postmenopausal endometrium as assessed by transvaginal ultrasonography and biopsy.[62b] In contrast, conjugated estrogens increased uterine volume and the incidence of endometrial hyperplasia and proliferative endometrium.[62b]

Interim results from the large Multiple Outcomes of Raloxifene Evaluation (MORE, n = 7705) in postmenopausal women with osteoporosis were recently reported.[63] Therapy with raloxifene 60 mg/day for 3 years significantly reduced the risk for vertebral fractures by 30% and 50% in women with and without pre-existing fractures, respectively, compared with calcium and vitamin D therapy (plus placebo) alone. As in the prevention study population, there was a significant increase in BMD (about 2 to 3% above baseline at the spine and hip) and a sustained reduction in markers of bone metabolism during raloxifene therapy.

Thus, the efficacy of raloxifene to reduce osteoporotic fractures – about the same as that of the potent antiresorptive alendronate – appears not to be reflected in its modest effects on spine

BMD; the mechanism for this remains unclear. The only adverse events thought to be associated with raloxifene in some patients in MORE were venous thromboembolism (see below), hot flashes and idiopathic leg cramps.

Short term effects of ERT/HRT to improve modestly mood and verbal memory in postmenopausal women have been demonstrated in some[64] but not all[65] randomised trials. Recently, the benefit of long term ERT/HRT on cognition as determined by some observational studies has been called into question.[66] Thus, confirmation of long term ERT/HRT effects on cognition await the results from controlled, clinical trials, such as the Heart and Estrogen/progestin Replacement Study (HERS) and Women's Health Initiative (WHI) trials.

The effect of SERMs on cognition and mood has been less extensively investigated. Preclinical data suggest that raloxifene and its analogues mimic estrogens in some respects but not others. For example, whereas estrogen increases hippocampal CA1 cell dendritic spine density and hypothalamic progesterone receptors in ovariectomised rats, a raloxifene analogue did not.[67] On the other hand, raloxifene increased hippocampal choline acetyltransferase activity and a raloxifene analogue increased hippocampal trkA gene expression in ovariectomised rats to approximately the same degree as estradiol and also produced a differential gene display pattern virtually identical to estrogen.[67,68] Raloxifene also induced neurite outgrowth in rat PC12 cells to an equal extent as estradiol.[69] A recent randomised trial of approximately 150 postmenopausal women with established osteoporosis indicated no measurable effects of raloxifene on mood or cognition after 1 year of treatment.[70] An extensive evaluation of cognition and neuropsychometric parameters in 7705 postmenopausal women with osteoporosis is being performed as part of the MORE trial. Six cognitive tests were administered, and cognitive decline was defined as change in score from baseline to 36 months in the worst 10th percentile. Three years of raloxifene therapy (combined 60mg and 120mg groups) did not affect overall cognitive scores in osteoporotic but otherwise healthy postmenopausal women. In women older than 70 years of age, raloxifene decreased the risk of decline in attention and memory, and improved attention and verbal memory performance.[70a]

In a 6-month randomised, placebo- and HRT-controlled trial, raloxifene lowered serum total and LDL-C comparably to continuous combined HRT (by about 11%) without significantly changing HDL-C or triglyceride levels.[71] The putative cardioprotective subfraction of HDL-C, known as HDL-C subfraction-2 was increased significantly by raloxifene, to about half the extent of HRT. Raloxifene also significantly lowered plasma fibrinogen by about 15% but did not change plasminogen activator inhibitor-1 (PAI-1) levels; in contrast, HRT affected fibrinogen only minimally and reduced PAI-1 significantly.[71] In the same study, HRT increased C-reactive protein levels by 84%, while raloxifene had no effect. Raloxifene and HRT both decreased serum fasting homocysteine levels similarly (6-8%).[71a]

Based on these favourable changes in these biochemical markers of cardiovascular risk, it might be expected that raloxifene and HRT would confer some protection against CHD. Recently, however, the negative results from HERS and 2-year interim results from WHI have raised doubts about a cardioprotective effect of HRT in postmenopausal women with established CHD;[72,72a]similarly, doubts will likely also exist for raloxifene until the CHD end-point results from raloxifene clinical trials such as Raloxifene Use for the Heart (RUTH) are available. In the interim, preclinical studies have yielded conflicting results, some indicating an ability of raloxifene to reduce aortic lipid accumulation and carotid intimal thickness in response to injury and one demonstrating no apparent effect of raloxifene on coronary artery plaque formation in primates.[73-75] The relevance of these findings to postmenopausal women will be known when outcome data from controlled clinical trials become available.[76,77]

The incidence of breast cancer was a defined secondary end-point of the MORE trial. After a median follow-up of 40 months, 40 cases of invasive breast cancer had been diagnosed (13 among pooled raloxifene 60 and 120 mg/day doses and 27 on placebo). Raloxifene reduced the incidence of invasive breast cancer by 76% (RR 0.24, 95% CI 0.13, 0.44) in postmenopausal women with osteoporosis. This reduction was driven by the significant 90% reduction in invasive estrogen-receptor positive breast cancers (RR 0.10, 95% CI 0.04, 0.24).[78]

From the same study, it was apparent that raloxifene, like tamoxifen and HRT, also increases the risk of venous thromboembolism by about 3-fold overall.[30,79] The risk appears to be highest soon after initiating therapy. Notably, venous thromboembolism is uncommon in generally healthy, postmenopausal women.

As mentioned previously, a raloxifene study which began in 1998 will assess CHD morbidity and mortality, among other end-points, in postmenopausal women at increased risk of cardiovascular disease (RUTH). A trial directly comparing raloxifene with tamoxifen for prevention of breast cancer in postmenopausal women at high risk (Study of Tamoxifen and Raloxifene, STAR) is currently enrolling. The total expected enrolment in RUTH and STAR is projected to be 10 000 and 22 000, respectively.

Another orally active benzothiophene, arzoxifene, which is as effective as but more potent than both raloxifene and Faslodex® as an ER antagonist in the rat endometrium,[80] and also more potent than raloxifene as an ER agonist on bone and serum lipids, is being evaluated clinically.[81] Arzoxifene has also been directly compared with lasofoxifene (a novel tetrahydronaphthalene in early clinical testing for osteoporosis) in the ovariectomised rat model. In these studies, arzoxifene had comparable maximal effects to lasofoxifene in the skeleton and on serum lipids but was significantly less stimulatory to the endometrium.[82] In a phase I clinical trial, arzoxifene 20 mg/day favourably altered biomarkers from biopsied breast tissue in 40 pre- and postmenopausal women after a mean of 17 days.[82a] In an ongoing phase II clinical trial, 92 patients (mean age 70 years) with locally advanced or metastatic breast cancer were randomised to receive arzoxifene 20 mg/day or 50 mg/day. Median time to progression was 10.4 months and 8.4 months for 20 and 50 mg/day doses, respectively; the investigator-determined objective response (CR+PR) rate was 34% and 36%, respectively.[82b] In a study of 32 patients with advanced or recurrent endometrial cancer that was potentially prostaglandin sensitive, arzoxifene resulted in 7 confirmed partial responses, 16 stable disease, and 9 progressive disease through up to 8 months of treatment.[82c] The most common adverse events in these trials were hot flashes, lymphopenia, anaemia and nausea, with no incidence of vaginal bleeding.[82b,c]

3. The Future of SERMs Research

What is the ideal SERM? If there is none today, how will we find one? These questions are now the focus of significant SERM research throughout the scientific community. We believe the answer to both questions is that there is not now, nor will there ever be, an ‘ideal’ SERM, just as there is no ideal cancer treatment nor antibiotic nor antihypertensive, etc. Undoubtedly, many SERMs will be developed in an attempt to meet a multitude of medical needs in both women and men. The SERMs currently targeting postmenopausal women are thus the archetypes for a rich category of drug therapy based on a single molecular target.

We have briefly reviewed the molecular basis for SERM tissue specificity. Each of the elements in the pathway to estrogen action is potentially subject to pharmacological intervention. Thus, the synthesis, metabolism and cellular (or nuclear) access of endogenous estrogens can be manipulated. ER ligands that preferentially bind to and/or activate one ER isoform over another may now be sought empirically via large scale screening. Small molecules that either interfere with or enhance interactions between ER and its co-activators/co-repressors are within reach of rational drug design. Similarly, molecules that selectively interfere with or enhance second messenger pathways that interact with and regulate ER action might prove useful. Which, if any, of these potential targets of SERM drug discovery will be successful clinically will not be known for several years. For now, postmenopausal women have a new choice for chronic disease prevention in raloxifene, and with that new choice, the scientific community has a strong impetus to expand their knowledge of ER and other nuclear receptors further.

Acknowledgements

The authors are indebted to Ms Erin Walls, ELS for her excellent technical assistance.

References

1. Sato M, Glasebrook AL, Bryant HU. Raloxifene: a selective estrogen receptor modulator. J Bone Miner Metab 1994; 12: S9-20
1a. Ray S, Dwivedy I. Development of estrogen antagonists as pharmaceutical agents. Adv Drug Res 1997; 29: 171-270
2. Stevenson J, Gaspard U, Avouac B, et al. Points to consider for the development of new indications for hormone replacement therapies and estrogen-like molecules. Climacteric 1998; 1: 12-7
3. Brzozowski AM, Pike ACW, Dauter Z, et al. Molecular basis of agonism and antagonism in the oestrogen receptor. Nature 1997; 389: 753-8
4. Grese TA, Sluka JP, Bryant HU, et al. Molecular determinants of tissue selectivity of estrogen receptor modulators. Proc Natl Acad Sci U S A 1997; 94: 14105-10
5. Katzenellenbogen JA, O'Malley BW, Katzenellenbogen BS. Tripartite steroid hormone receptor pharmacology: interaction with multiple effector sites as a basis for the cell- and promoter-specific action of these hormones. Mol Endocrinol 1996; 10: 119-31
6. McDonnell DP, Norris JD. Analysis of the molecular pharmacology of estrogen receptor agonists and antagonists provides insights into the mechanism of action of estrogen in bone. Osteoporos Int 1997; 7 (1 Suppl.): 29-34
7. Jensen EV, Jacobson HI. Basic guides to the mechanism of estrogen action. In: Pincus G, editor. Recent progress in hormone research: The Proceedings of the 1961 Laurentian Hormone Conference. New York: Academic Press, 1962: (18) 387-414
8. Gorski J, Toft D, Shyamala G, et al. Hormone receptors: studies on the interaction of estrogen with the uterus. In: Astwood EB, editor. Recent progress in hormone research: The Proceedings of the 1961 Laurentian Hormone Conference. New York: Academic Press, 1968: (24) 45-80
9. Anstead GM, Carlson KE, Katzenellenbogen JA. The estradiol pharmacophore: ligand structure-estrogen receptor binding affinity relationships and a model for the receptor binding site. Steroids 1997; 62: 268-303
10. Giguere V, Tremblay A, Tremblay GB. Estrogen receptor β: re-evaluation of estrogen and antiestrogen signalling. Steroids 1998; 63: 335-9
11. Murphy LC, Leygue E, Dotzlaw H, et al. Oestrogen receptor variants and mutations in human breast cancer. Ann Med 1997; 29: 221-34
12. Tzukerman M, Esty A, Santiso-Mere D, et al. Human estrogen receptor transactivational capacity is determined by both cellular and promoter context and mediated by two functionally distinct intramolecular regions. Mol Endocrinol 1994; 8 (1): 21-30
13. Danielian PS, White R, Lees JA, et al. Identification of a conserved region required for hormone dependent transcriptional activation by steroid hormone receptors [published erratum appears in EMBO J 1992; 11: 2366]. EMBO J 1992; 11: 1025-33
14. Norris JD, Fan D, Kerner SA, et al. Identification of a third autonomous activation domain within the human estrogen receptor. Mol Endocrinol 1997; 11: 747-54
15. Berry M, Metzger D, Chambon P. Role of the two activating domains of the oestrogen receptor in the cell-type and promoter-context dependent agonistic activity of the anti-oestrogen 4-hydroxytamoxifen. EMBO J 1990; 9: 2811-8
16. McDonnell DP, Clemm DL, Hermann T, et al. Analysis of estrogen receptor function in vitro reveals three distinct classes of antiestrogens. Mol Endocrinol 1995; 9: 659-69
17. Feng W, Ribeiro RCJ, Wagner RL, et al. Hormone-dependent coactivator binding to a hydrophobic cleft on nuclear receptors. Science 1998; 280: 1747-9

18. Levenson AS, Jordan VC. The key to the antiestrogenic mechanism of raloxifene is amino acid 351 (aspartate) in the estrogen receptor. Cancer Res 1998; 58(9): 1872-5
19. Yang NN, Venugopalan M, Hardikar S, et al. Identification of an estrogen response element activated by metabolites of 17beta-estradiol and raloxifene [published erratum appears in Science 1997; 275: 1249]. Science 1996; 273: 1222-5
20. Elgort MG, Zou A, Marschke KB, et al. Estrogen and estrogen receptor antagonists stimulate transcription from the human retinoic acid receptor-α-1 promoter via a novel sequence. Mol Endocrinol 1996; 10: 477-87
21. Webb P, Lopez GN, Uht RM, et al. Tamoxifen activation of the estrogen receptor/AP-1 pathway: potential origin for the cell-specific estrogen-like effects of antiestrogens. Mol Endocrinol 1995; 9: 443-56
22. Paech K, Webb P, Kuiper GGJM, et al. Differential ligand activation of estrogen receptors ER alpha and ER beta at AP1 sites. Science 1997; 277: 1508-10
23. Enmark E, Pelto-Huikko M, Grandien K, et al. Human estrogen receptor β-gene structure, chromosomal localization, and expression pattern. J Clin Endocrinol Metab 1997; 82: 4258-68
24. White R, Parker MG. Molecular mechanisms of steroid hormone action. Endocr Rel Cancer 1998; 5: 1-14
25. Robyr D, Wolffe AP. Hormone action and chromatin remodelling. Cell Mol Life Sci 1998; 54: 113-24
26. Bedford GR, Richardson DN. Preparation and identification of cis and trans isomers of a substituted triarylethylene. Nature 1966; 212: 733-4
27. Harper MJ, Walpole AL. Contrasting endocrine activities of cis and trans isomers in a series of substituted triphenylethylenes. Nature 1966; 212: 87
28. Cole MP, Jones CT, Todd ID. A new anti-oestrogenic agent in late breast cancer. An early clinical appraisal of ICI46474. Br J Cancer 1971; 25: 270-5
29. Early Breast Cancer Trialists' Collaborative Group. Tamoxifen for early breast cancer: an overview of the randomised trials. Lancet 1998; 351: 1451-67
30. Fisher B, Dignam J, Bryant J, et al. Five versus more than five years of tamoxifen therapy for breast cancer patients with negative lymph nodes and estrogen receptor-positive tumors. J Natl Cancer Inst 1996; 88: 1529-42
31. Resch A, Biber E, Seifer M, et al. Evidence that tamoxifen preserves bone density in late postmenopausal women with breast cancer. Acta Oncologica 1998; 37: 661-4
32. Marttunen MB, Hietanen P, Tiitinen A, et al. Comparison of effects of tamoxifen and toremifene on bone biochemistry and bone mineral density in postmenopausal breast cancer patients. J Clin Endocrinol Metab 1998; 83: 1158-62
33. McDonald CC, Alexander FE, Whyte BW, et al. Cardiac and vascular morbidity in women receiving adjuvant tamoxifen for breast cancer in a randomised trial. The Scottish Cancer Trials Breast Group. BMJ 1995; 311: 977-80
34. Grey AB, Stapleton JP, Evans MC, et al. The effect of the antiestrogen tamoxifen on bone mineral density in normal late postmenopausal women. Am J Med 1995; 99: 636-41
35. Powles TJ, Hickish T, Kanis JA, et al. Effect of tamoxifen on bone mineral density measured by dual-energy x-ray absorptiometry in healthy premenopausal and postmenopausal women. J Clin Oncol 1996; 14: -84
36. Chang J, Powles TJ, Ashley SE, et al. The effect of tamoxifen and hormone replacement therapy on serum cholesterol, bone mineral density and coagulation factors in healthy postmenopausal women participating in a randomised, controlled tamoxifen prevention study. Ann Oncol 1996; 7: 671-5
37. Gotfredsen A, Christiansen C, Palshof T. The effect of tamoxifen on bone mineral content in premenopausal women with breast cancer. Cancer 1984; 53: 853-7
38. Fisher B, Costantino JP, Wickerham DL, et al. Tamoxifen for prevention of breast cancer: report of the National Surgical Adjuvant Breast and Bowel Project P-1 Study. J Natl Cancer Inst 1998; 90 (18): 1371-88
39. Veronesi U, Maisonneuve P, Costa A, et al. Prevention of breast cancer with tamoxifen: preliminary findings from the Italian randomised trial among hysterectomised women. Italian Tamoxifen Prevention Study. Lancet 1998; 352: 93-7
40. Powles T, Eeles R, Ashley S, et al. Interim analysis of the incidence of breast cancer in the Royal Marsden Hospital tamoxifen randomised chemoprevention trial. Lancet 1998; 352: 98-101
41. Ray A. Side effects of tamoxifen are distressing and common [letter]. BMJ 1996; 313: 1484
42. Love RR, Cameron L, Connell BL, et al. Symptoms associated with tamoxifen treatment in postmenopausal women. Arch Intern Med 1991; 151: 1842-7
43. Gershanovich M, Hayes DF, Ellmen J, et al. High-dose toremifene *vs* tamoxifen in postmenopausal advanced breast cancer. Oncology 1997; 11: 29-36
44. Saarto T, Blomqvist C, Ehnholm C, et al. Antiatherogenic effects of adjuvant antiestrogens: a randomized trial comparing the effects of tamoxifen and toremifene on plasma lipid levels in postmenopausal women with node-positive breast cancer. J Clin Oncol 1996; 14: 429-33
45. Marttunen MB, Hietanen P, Tiitinen A, et al. Comparison of effects of tamoxifen and toremifene on bone biochemistry and bone mineral density in postmenopausal breast cancer patients. J Clin Endocrinol Metab 1998; 83: 1158-62
46. Rauschning W, Pritchard KI. Droloxifene, a new antiestrogen: its role in metastatic breast cancer. Breast Cancer Res Treat 1994: 31: 83-94
47. Press Release of Ligand Pharmaceuticals Incorporated. Pfizer to Focus on Lasoxifene - CP336,156 - for Osteoporosis and Breast Cancer; Ligand to Receive Milestones and Royalties on Further Development. BW Health Wire Issued December 23, 1999, San Diego, Business Editors/Health & Medical Writers

47a. Smith Kline Press Release: SmithKline Beecham drops idoxifene for osteoporosis. Scrip 1999; 2431-21

48. Weiss S, Mulder H, Chesnut C, et al. Idoxifene reduces bone turnover in osteopenic postmenopausal women [abstract]. 80th Annual Meeting of the Endocrine Society. The Endocrine Society Program & Abstracts: 1998 June 24-27; New Orleans (LA), 403
49. Fleischer AC, Wheeler JE, Yeh IT, et al. Sonographic assessment of the endometrium in osteopenic postmenopausal women treated with idoxifene. J Ultrasound Med 1999; 18: 503-12

50. SmithKline Beecham. SmithKline Beecham emphasises research and development strengths after failed merger talks [press release]. Scrip 1998 April 22
51. Kamboj VP, Ray S, Dhawan B. Centcroman. Drugs Today 1992; 28: 227-32
52. Salman M, Ray S, Anand N, et al. Studies in antifertility agents. Stereoselective binding of d- and 1-centchromans to estrogen receptors and their antifertility activity. J Med Chem 1986; 29: 1801-3
53. Skrumsager BK, Kiehr B, Bjarnason K. Levormeloxifene: escalating single oral doses in healthy postmenopausal women [abstract]. J Bone Miner Res 1997; 12: S346
54. Skrumsager BK, Kiehr B, Bjarnason K. Levormeloxifene: safety and pharmacokinetics after multiple dosing of fifty-six postmenopausal women [abstract]. J Bone Miner Res 1997; 12: S346
55. Bjarnason K, Skrumsager BK, Kiehr B. Levormeloxifene, a new partial estrogen receptor agonist demonstrates antiresorptive and antiatherogenic properties in postmenopausal women [abstract]. J Bone Miner Res 1997; 12: S346
56. Sacks FM, Pfeffer MA, Moye LA, et al. The effect of pravastatin on coronary events after myocardial infarction in patients with average cholesterol levels. Cholesterol and Recurrent Events Trial investigators. N Engl J Med 1996; 335: 1001-9
57. Kannel WB, Wolf PA, Castelli WP, et al. Fibrinogen and risk of cardiovascular disease: The Framingham Study. JAMA 1987; 258: 1183-6
58. Novo Nordisk, Bagsvaerd, Denmark. Novo Nordisk levormeloxifene phase 2 clinical trial: Novo Nordisk presents phase 2 data on levormeloxifene to clinical investigators [press release]. PRNewswire 1998 June 19
59. Glasebrook AL, Phillips DL, Sluka JP. Multiple binding-sites for the antiestrogen raloxifene (LY156758) [abstract no. 607]. J Bone Miner Res 1993; 8: S268
60. Gize EA, Venugopalan M, Glasebrook AL, et al. Characterization of raloxifene binding and transactivation properties of the estrogen receptor-beta (ER beta) [abstract]. J Bone Miner Res 1997; 12: S460
61. Heaney RP, Draper MW. Raloxifene mimics estrogen in human bone remodelling kinetics. J Bone Miner Res 1996; 11 (1 Suppl.): S446
62. Cohen FJ, Lu Y. Characterization of hot flashes reported by healthy postmenopausal women receiving raloxifene or placebo during osteoporosis prevention trials. Maturitas 2000; 34: 65-73

62a. Cohen FJ, Watts S, Shah A, et al. Uterine effects of three-year raloxifene therapy in postmenopausal women under age 60. Obstet Gynecol 2000; 95: 104-10

62b. Goldstein SR, Scheele WH, Rajagopalan SK, et al. A 12-month comparative study of raloxifene, estrogen, and placebo on the postmenopausal endometrium. Obstet Gynecol 2000; 95: 95-103

63. Ettinger B, Black DM, Mitlak BH, et al. Reduction of vertebral fracture risk in postmenopausal women with osteoporosis treated with raloxifene: results from a 3-year randomized clinical trial. JAMA 1999; 282: 637-45
64. Phillips SM, Sherwin BB. Effects of estrogen on memory function in surgically menopausal women. Psychoneuroendocrinology 1992; 17 (5): 485-95
65. Polo-Kantola P, Portin R, Polo O, et al. The effect of short-term estrogen replacement therapy on cognition: a randomized, double-blind, cross-over trial in postmenopausal women. Obstet Gynecol 1998; 91 (3): 459-66
66. Yaffe K, Sawaya G, Lieberburg I, et al. Estrogen therapy in postmenopausal women. JAMA 1998; 279: 688-95
67. Bryant HU, Bales KR, Paul SM, et al. Estrogen agonist effects of selective estrogen receptor modulators in ovariectomized rat brain [abstract]. Soc Neurosci Abstr 1997; 23: 2377
68. Wu X, Glinn MA, Ostrowski NL, et al. Raloxifene and estradiol benzoate both fully restore hippocampal choline acetyltransferase activity in ovariectomized rats. Brain Research 1999; 847: 98-104
69. Nilsen J, Mor G, Naftolin F. Raloxifene induces neurite outgrowth in estrogen receptor positive PC12 cells. Menopause 1998; 5 (4): 211-6
70. Nickelsen T, Lufkin EG, Riggs BL, et al. Raloxifene hydrochloride, a selective estrogen receptor modulator: safety assessment of effects on cognitive function and mood in postmenopausal women. Psychoneuroendocrinology 1999; 24: 115-28

70a. Krueger KA, Yaffe K, Sarkar S, et al. Effects of raloxifene on cognitive function in postmenopausal women without dementia [abstract no. P389]. Final Program, American Geriatrics Society/American Federation for Aging Research, 2000 Annual Scientific Meeting; 2000 May 17-21: Nashville, TN: 170

71. Walsh BW, Kuller LH, Wild RA, et al. Effects of raloxifene on serum lipids and coagulation factors in healthy postmenopausal women. JAMA 1998; 279: 1445-51

71a. Walsh B, Paul S, Wild RA, et al. Effects of hormone replacement therapy and raloxifene on C-reactive protein and homocysteine in postmenopausal women: a randomized, controlled trial. J Endocrinol Metab 2000; 85: 214-8

72. Hulley S, Grady D, Bush T, Heart and Estrogen/progestin Replacement Study (HERS) Research Group, et al. Randomized trial of estrogen plus progestin for secondary prevention of coronary heart disease in postmenopausal women. JAMA 1998; 280: 605-13

72a. WHI Press Release. Press Release of the Women's Health Initiative (WHI) Study. Hormone replacement study finds slight rise in heart problems. The Washington Post via Dow Vision A Section, A08, 2000

73. Bjarnason NH, Haarbo J, Byrjalsen I, et al. Raloxifene inhibits aortic accumulation of cholesterol in ovariectomized, cholesterol-fed rabbits. Circulation 1997; 96 (6): 1964-9
74. Kauffman RF, Bean JS, Bensch WR. Effects of estrogen and raloxifene, a selective estrogen receptor modulator, in animal models of vascular injury. In: Rubanyi GM, Kauffman R, editors. Estrogen and the vessel wall. Amsterdam: Harwood Academic Publishers, 1998
75. Clarkson TB, Anthony MS, Jerome CP. Lack of effect of raloxifene on coronary artery atherosclerosis of postmenopausal monkeys. J Clin Endocrinol Metab 1998; 83: 721-6
76. Bryant HU, Kauffman RF, Iversen P, et al. Comment on lack of effect of raloxifene on coronary artery atherosclerosis of postmenopausal monkeys [letter]. J Clin Endocrinol Metab 1998; 83 (8): 3001-2

77. Clarkson TB, Anthony MS. Lack of effect of raloxifene on coronary atherosclerosis of postmenopausal monkeys: authors' response [letter]. J Clin Endocrinol Metab 1998; 83 (8): 3002-4
78. Cummings S, Eckert S, Krueger K, et al. The effect of raloxifene on risk of breast cancer in postmenopausal women. JAMA 1999; 281: 2189-97
79. Castellsague J, Perez-Gutthann S, Garcia Rodriguez LA. Recent epidemiological studies of the association between hormone replacement therapy and venous thromboembolism: a review. Drug Saf 1998; 18: 117-23
80. Bryant HU, Glasebrook AL, Knadler MP, et al. A highly potent orally active selective estrogen receptor modulator [abstract]. 79th Annual Meeting of the Endocrine Society. The Endocrine Society Program & Abstracts: 1997 June 11-14; Minneapolis (MN), 548
81. Sato M, Turner CH, Wang T, et al. LY353381.HCl: a novel raloxifene analog with improved SERM potency and efficacy in vivo. J Pharmacol Exp Ther 1998; 287: 1-7
82. Cole HW, Adrian MD, Shetler PK, et al. Comparative pharmacology of high potency selective estrogen receptor modulators (SERMs) [abstract]. J Bone Miner Res 1997; 12: S349
82a. Fabian CJ, Kimler BF, Anderson J, et al. Phase I biomarker and toxicity evaluation of LY353381 (a 3rd generation selective estrogen receptor modulator, SERM) in breast cancer. Thirty-Sixth Annual Meeting of the American Society of Clinical Oncology Program Proceedings; 2000 May 20-23: Baltimore, MD: Lippincott Williams & Wilkins, 2000: 290
82b. Llombart-Cussac A, Bellet M, Guillem-Porta V, et al. Efficacy and safety of two doses of the selective estrogen receptor modulator (SERM) LY353381 in locally advanced or metastatic breast cancer (Lambc) – a randomized double-blind phase 2 study. Thirty-Sixth Annual Meeting of the American Society of Clinical Oncology Program Proceedings; 2000 May 20-23: Baltimore, MD: Lippincott Williams & Wilkins, 2000: 6090
82c. Klinj J. Multicentre phase II study of the selective estrogen receptor modulator (SERM) LY353381 in advanced or recurrent cancer – objective responses in progestagen sensitive patients (PTS). Thirty-Sixth Annual Meeting of the American Society of Clinical Oncology Program Proceedings; 2000 May 20-23: Baltimore, MD: Lippincott Williams & Wilkins, 2000: 1527

Correspondence: Dr *Bruce H. Mitlak*, Eli Lilly and Company, Lilly Corporate Center DC2244, Indianapolis, IN 46285, USA. Dr *Frederic J. Cohen*, RW Johnson Pharmaceutical Research Institute, 920 Route 202, Raritan, NJ 08869, USA.
E-mail: b.mitlak@lilly.com, fcohen1@prius.jnj.com

Osteoporosis as a Candidate for Disease Management

Epidemiological and Cost-of-Illness Considerations

David Torgerson[1] and *Cyrus Cooper*[2]

1 National Primary Care Research and Development, Centre for Health Economics, University of York, York, England

2 Medical Research Council Environmental Epidemiology Unit, Southampton General Hospital, Southampton, England

Osteoporosis is a skeletal disease characterised by low bone mass and microarchitectural deterioration of bone tissue with a consequent increase in bone fragility and susceptibility to fracture.[1] The disorder is a major health problem through its relationship with these fractures which typically occur at 3 skeletal sites: the hip, wrist and vertebra. The advent of bone densitometry has shown that fractures at other sites (proximal humerus, pelvis, rib, clavicle and distal femur) are also associated with low bone density. One-third of the population aged >65 years fall annually and of these, 1% will fracture a bone.[2]

1. Osteoporotic Fractures

1.1 Hip Fracture

Hip fracture is the most severe osteoporotic fracture. Most hip fractures follow a fall from the standing position, although they are known to occur spontaneously. Overall, 90% of hip fractures occur among people aged 50 years and over, and 80% occur in women.[3] The average age at which hip fractures occur in the UK is 79 years. This pattern is similar in most Western populations.

Hip fractures are seasonal; they occur more frequently during winter in temperate countries, but the majority of fractures are from falls indoors and are not related to slipping on icy pavements.[4] The seasonality of hip fractures is as marked in the southern hemisphere as it is in Europe and North America.[5] Explanations for the seasonality of hip fractures include abnormal neuromuscular function at lower temperatures and a reduction in sunlight exposure during winter. Age- and sex-adjusted hip fracture rates are generally higher in White than in Black or Asian populations,[6] although urbanisation in certain parts of Africa has led to higher hip fracture rates. Furthermore, the pronounced female preponderance of hip fractures observed in White populations is not seen among Black or Asian populations, in which rates for men and women are similar.[7]

Geographic variation in hip fracture has been studied extensively in the US, Sweden and the UK. In the US, there is a north to south gradient with highest rates of fracture in the south-east. Other factors that seem to have a detrimental effect on hip fracture rate include socioeconomic deprivation, decreased sunlight exposure and fluoridated water supply.[8]

Living in a rural community appears to be a protective factor in Sweden and the UK (East Anglia).[3] Thus, demographic changes over the next 60 years will lead to huge increases in the number of hip fractures requiring medical care. In Europe, the growth of the elderly portion of the population will increase fracture numbers to 80% by the year 2025.[9] This increase will be even more dramatic in Asia. Superimposed on these changes in population age structure are secular trends in the age-specific incidence of hip fracture, which have increased in recent decades.[3] However, the most recent data shows a slowing of this increase.

1.2 Vertebral Fracture

Epidemiological information on vertebral fractures has been hampered by the absence of a universally accepted definition of vertebral deformity from lateral thoracolumbar x-rays and because a substantial proportion of vertebral deformities are asymptomatic. The application of recently developed definitions to various population samples in the US has permitted estimation of the incidence of new vertebral fractures in the general population.[10]

The incidence of all vertebral deformities among postmenopausal White women has been estimated to be around three times that of hip fracture. However, the incidence of clinically ascertained vertebral deformities is around 30% of this total figure. The overall age-adjusted female to male incidence ratio for these deformities is 1.9. The most frequent vertebral levels involved are the weakest regions in the spine: T8, T12 and L1. Vertebral fracture rarely leads to hospitalisation in the UK; as few as 2% of patients may be admitted. However, clinical coding inadequacies remain a source of underestimation for this figure. The economic burden of vertebral fracture is mainly due to the cost of outpatient care, the provision of nursing care and the loss of working days. Of those patients seeking medical attention, at least 80% had a grade 2 deformity or above. In women, vertebral fracture is only associated with minor or moderate trauma (90%), whilst in men, 37% may be associated with significant trauma.

1.3 Wrist Fracture

Wrist fractures display a different pattern of occurrence to hip or spine fractures. In White women, wrist fracture rates increase linearly between the ages of 40 and 65 years and then stabilise. In White men, the incidence remains constant between the ages of 20 and 80 years. The reason for the plateau in female incidence remains obscure, but it may relate to a change in the pattern of falling with advancing age. As in the case of hip fracture, the majority of wrist fractures occur in women and around 50% occur among women aged 65 years and over. The winter peak in wrist fracture incidence is even greater than that seen for hip fracture.

Some of the differences in timing of the different types of osteoporotic fracture may be due to the loss of different types of bone. Trabecular bone is particularly subject to estrogen deficiency after the menopause, and it has been suggested that a specific type of osteoporosis (type 1) occurs in postmenopausal women.[11] Colles' fracture is due to a combination of rapid trabecular loss in the distal forearm and trauma to this area, whilst vertebral compression of fractures are often associated with minimal trauma. Typically, patients aged in their 60s present with back pain or kyphosis ('Dowager's Hump').

Table I. Impact of osteoporotic fractures in men and women in the UK[13]

	Hip	Spine	Wrist
Lifetime risk of osteoporotic fracture (%)			
women (aged 50y)	14	11	13
men (aged 50y)	3	2	2
Mean age at which osteoporotic fracture occurs (y)	79	67	65
Mortality from osteoporotic fractures (relative survival)	0.83	0.82	1.00
Functional impairment caused by osteoporotic fractures (%)	30	10	10
Cost	All sites combined = £942 million/year (1995-1996)		

Type 2 osteoporosis occurs in men and women over the age of 70 years and affects cortical and trabecular bone. It is in this age group that we see a much increased risk of hip fracture. Low dietary calcium, vitamin D and sunlight deficiency, calcium malabsorption and decreased renal conversion of 25-hydroxyvitamin D to 1,25-hydroxyvitamin D all contribute to secondary hyperparathyroidism and an increased but inadequate osteoblast response to increased osteoclast resorption.

Finally, osteoporosis may occur as a consequence of the use of corticosteroids, thyrotoxicosis or prolonged immobilisation. These risk factors represent potent opportunities for prevention, yet their understanding the understanding of these factors is poorly developed.

2. The Burden of Osteoporotic Fracture

Table I shows the impact of osteoporotic fractures in men and women in the UK. The lifetime risk of hip fractures among 50-year-old women is 14%, and the risk among 50-year-old men is 3%. In contrast, the risk among White women and men is 11% and 2% respectively, for clinically diagnosed spine fractures, and 13% and 2% respectively, for wrist fractures. On average, hip fractures occur around 15 years later than spine and wrist fractures. They are also attended by a greater risk of serious functional impairment and institutionalisation. The total cost of osteoporosis is difficult to assess because it includes acute hospital care, loss of working days and long term residential care. In England and Wales the total cost was estimated in 1994 at £742 million[12] and this figure will increase as the proportion of elderly in society rises.

Extrapolating UK incidence rates for these fractures to a typical general practice listing of 2000 patients, the annual incidence rate of all osteoporotic fractures will be 7 to 8 per year. These can be broken down as 2 to 3 hip fractures, 2 wrist fractures, 2 clinically diagnosed vertebral deformities and a further 5 patients with newly detected vertebral deformities that are silent. Table II shows the number of men and women with prevalent vertebral deformities in this typical practice. The frequency rises from 2 men and 4 women in the 45 to 54 year age band up to 14 men and 7 women aged ≥85 years.

Table II. Prevalence of vertebral deformity in men and women in the UK. The figures were derived by applying the UK prevalence rate to the demography of a typical general practice of 2000 patients

Age (y)	Number of individuals with vertebral deformity	
	Men	Women
45-54	2	4
55-64	4	6
65-74	7	11
75-84	12	20
≥85	14	7
All	29	48

The burden of osteoporosis can also be characterised by examining the prevalence of low bone density in the general population. Recently, an expert panel convened by the WHO devised an operational definition of osteoporosis[14] in which low bone density (or osteopenia) was defined by a bone mineral density (BMD) >1 standard deviation (SD) below the young normal mean, but <2.5 SD below. Women with BMD levels >2.5 SD below the young normal mean are defined as having osteoporosis. If an individual with BMD below this threshold also has a fragility fracture, they fulfil the definition of having established osteoporosis. Table III shows the prevalence of osteoporosis among women in the UK using the WHO definition.[14] In the age group 50 to 59 years, the frequency of osteoporosis at the hip only is 3.9% and at any site it is 14.8%. This rises to 47.5% and 70%, respectively, in women aged ≥80 years.

Table III. Prevalence of osteoporosis using the WHO definition: data for women in the UK[14]

Age	Osteoporosis	
	any site (%)	hip only (%)
50-59	14.8	3.9
60-69	21.6	8.0
70-79	38.5	24.5
≥80	70	47.5

3. Preventive Strategies

As bone loss with age is a universal phenomenon, prevention of osteoporosis is far better than attempting to treat the disorder once established. Two preventive strategies may be used: firstly, the treatment of individuals at high risk and; secondly, public health measures to shift the bone density distribution of the entire population. To achieve a 20% reduction in fracture risk, an attempt could be made to measure and effectively treat the 17% of the population at highest risk, or move the mean population bone density by around 3% in a beneficial direction. Peak bone mass, a main determinant of bone strength, can be influenced at different times throughout life by environmental factors. These include weight bearing/physical activity, dietary calcium intake and avoidance of tobacco and heavy alcohol consumption. These factors are all useful in the population-based approach; however, there is an absence of data from randomised controlled trials supporting the effectiveness of any of these strategies directly against fracture.

The more widespread availability of noninvasive techniques or the measurement of bone density and of drugs which retard bone loss, support the implementation of an individually-based preventive approach to accompany the population strategy. Bone densitometry provides a useful measure of future fracture risk and, although population based screening of peri-menopausal women cannot at present be justified, clinical indications for bone densitometry have been delineated for settings in which the result obtained will influence the management of individual patients. These include the presence of strong or multiple risk factors, radiological evidence of osteopenia and/or vertebral deformity, and a previous history of low trauma fractures of the limbs. Once measurements have been made, therapeutic agents may be used as indicated. Broadly, a treatment can be categorised as those drugs that prevent bone resorption and those that provide bone growth. Of the former, estrogen, calcium and vitamin D have a place to play in both primary and secondary prevention.

Estrogen therapy, or hormone replacement therapy (HRT), is now increasingly taken after the menopause, though its use decreases as women enter their 60s. Its other beneficial effect is on the cardiovascular system as well as on bone, but it may increase the risk of breast cancer in some patients. HRT acts to retard the rate of bone loss during the years it is taken, but the duration of treatment remains a problem. The Framingham Study examined this issue[15] and found that women in Framingham under the age of 75 years, who had taken long term estrogen therapy, had a bone mineral density higher than those who had not, although in those women over 75 years old there was little difference. This may be because estrogen withdrawal is followed by rapid bone loss. Bone mineral density is estimated to decrease by 2% per year in the first 5 years after the menopause and then by 1% per year, leading to a bone mineral density loss of approximately 30% between the ages of 50 to 80 years. Possible treatment options are to continue HRT indefinitely (which can be a compliance problem), to give treatment to only those women who have had a fracture or to start HRT later in life. However, taking HRT for 10 years, does not seem to be the complete answer. While the current focus of preventive strategies has been the early postmenopausal years in women, this is likely to shift to later ages for several reasons. Firstly, prospective data suggest that age-related bone loss continues throughout later life. Secondly, fracture incidence rises steeply with age; the cost-effectiveness of treatments will be maximised closer to the time when fractures occur. Finally, bone densitometry predicts fractures equally as well at age ≥75 years as at 65 years.

For age-related bone loss, calcium absorption is often blunted and, theoretically, calcium seems a suitable treatment option in the elderly who may be calcium depleted for several reasons. Dawson-Hughes et al.[16] studied a group of women for at least 5 years postmenopause whose normal calcium intake was approximately 400 mg/day; the study showed a beneficial effect of a 500 mg/day supplement. A further study of postmenopausal women taking supplements of 1000 mg/day also showed calcium slowed bone loss and nonrandomised clinical studies show calcium-supplemented patients have fewer fractures.[17] A study of calcium and vitamin D supplementation given to elderly women, resident in a French nursing home, showed higher femoral bone density and lower fracture rates in the treated groups,[18] whereas a study of vitamin D alone given to an elderly, noninstitutionalised population showed an increase in femoral bone density but no decreased fracture rate.

Bisphosphonates, in addition to calcitonin, anabolic steroids and low dose sodium fluoride tend to be reserved for secondary prevention in patients in whom a fracture has already occurred. Bisphosphonates are synthetic analogues of pyrophosphates. They inhibit osteoblast activity by binding to the hydroxyapatite crystals of bone absorption surfaces. One of the concerns of these drugs is that they are retained in the skeleton for up to 10 years and may therefore impair the ability to repair microfractures. Low dose intermittent cyclical administration of etidronate (etidronic acid) with calcium is widely used to treat vertebral osteoporosis; this has been shown to decrease fracture rates and increase bone density.[19,20] Newer bisphosphonates have also been shown to be effective in treating patients with established osteoporosis.[21]

The following treatment options are also occasionally used in the UK. Calcitonin has been shown to produce a small increase in bone mineral density and has the advantage of a centrally acting analgesic effect, but it has the disadvantages of being expensive and requiring administration by subcutaneous injection. Now that intranasal preparations are available its use may increase. Fluoride has been shown to increase bone density in two large randomised trials in the US, but unfortunately this does not correlate with decreased fracture rate.[22,23] Finally, anabolic steroids have been used in the frail elderly patient with osteoporosis to increase bone formation and muscle mass, but metabolic adverse effects prevent their long term use.

4. Costs of Osteoporotic Fracture

Osteoporotic fractures are expensive in financial terms; however, quantifying this cost is difficult for a number of reasons. For example, while the immediate treatment costs of hip fracture are almost entirely hospital-based, many survivors of hip fracture will require ongoing treatment and support after discharge from hospital.

In 1994, the cost of osteoporotic fractures for the UK only was estimated as being £742 million.[24] However, this figure was derived using US estimates of length of nursing home stay after hip fracture, which may not be applicable to the UK. This figure is substantially greater than another estimate of £288 million, or £5000 per hip fracture, which was based only on hospital costs for the UK.[25] A more recent estimate of the costs of osteoporosis for the UK was given as approximately £942 million for 1995 to 1996.[26]

Although osteoporosis is associated with a large financial cost, quantifying this as a total cost of illness is controversial amongst health economists.[27] Cost of illness studies do not tend to be helpful in deciding whether preventing a particularly costly disease is actually cost effective. Indeed, the inappropriate use of these studies may divert resources away from diseases which can be easily and cost effectively treated to those which are expensive but have a poor clinical outcome no matter how effectively treated.

5. Economic Considerations In the Prevention of Osteoporotic Fractures

A recent review has identified more than 20 economic evaluations on methods of preventing osteoporosis.[28] Most of the studies concentrate on evaluating the use of HRT for the prevention of fractures. The general conclusions of the studies are that for women with menopausal symptoms, HRT was a relatively cost-effective intervention. Hence, the cost per quality-adjusted life-year (QALY) gained ranged from $US3481 to $US22 656 in 1995. However, for women with no menopausal symptoms the results are less clear.[29] Under some assumptions, for example, no cardiovascular protection and a loss of QALYs due to breast cancer effects, HRT produces no net benefit for asymptomatic women. On the other hand, given more favourable cardiovascular assumptions and a lesser effect on breast cancer risk, there is a net benefit, however, the cost-effectiveness ratios are still greater than those for treating symptomatic women: range $US28 647 to $US75 993 in 1995. For women with menopausal symptoms, HRT was relatively cost effective with a cost per QALY ranging from $US3481 to $US22 656 (assuming 1990 $US prices). However, for asymptomatic women the results were more equivocal with costs per QALYs. Generally, targeting therapy improves the cost effectiveness ratios.[29]

All evaluations published since 1990 have assumed that the prevention method would consist of postmenopausal HRT for between 5 to 10 years starting soon after the menopause. However, recent evidence suggest that HRT needs to be taken for life to have a fracture protective effect.[30] Furthermore, economic evaluations published since 1990 have reached the consistent conclusion that intervening later on in the disease cycle will be more cost effective than intervening at the menopause.[28,29] Therefore, it seems clear that osteoporotic fractures are most cost effectively treated if therapy is given close to the age when fracture events are most likely to occur, i.e. in the seventh or eighth decades of life. Tosteson and colleagues[31] noted that targeting HRT using BMD measurements produced a cost per QALY of between $US11 700 and $US22 100 in 1990 (depending on which BMD value was chosen) compared with universal treatment which produced a marginal cost per QALY of $US349 000.

In general, modelling studies with respect to HRT can be divided into HRT and non-HRT analyses. Because of the diverse effects of HRT, modelling studies will always contain considerable uncertainty even if good trial data are available. Therefore, the anti-fracture effects of HRT as well as its effects on the breast, cardiovascular system and menopausal symptoms require inclusion in the model. In contrast, modelling the effects of, for example, a bisphosphonate is relatively straightforward as its only known effects are on bone; this considerably reduces the amount of uncertainty within any model.

Which therapy is the most cost effective is unclear as, to date, there has been no economic evaluation has been published which has used cost effectiveness and quality of life data from a clinical trial. Therefore, all the evaluations to date are modelling studies. Whilst modelling studies are important, they are no substitute for using data from trials as cost data suffers the same problem of confounding as does effectiveness data. Therefore, cost effectiveness judgements, at present, tend to rely heavily on the acquisition costs of various treatments. For example, an economic evaluation of the different treatments available to prevent vertebral fractures made the assumption that nonacquisition, or follow-up, costs were similar regardless of whether a patient was given HRT, bisphosphonates or any other therapy.[32] Clearly this may not be true.

One treatment which is likely to be highly cost effective is the use of hip protectors[33,34] particularly among men and women who have already sustained a hip fracture. Such protectors are cheap, highly effective and, for patients who have already sustained a hip fracture, very cost effective as such patients are likely to be compliant and are at an extremely high risk of sustaining a second fracture.[35] A recent economic evaluation suggested that even with compliance rates as low as 10% hip protectors appeared cost saving.[36]

Most pharmaceutical treatments, due to their high cost, will almost always need targeting towards highest risk groups either by the presence of a multitude of strong clinical risk factors or some form of measurement of bone mass. To achieve risk stratification, the cheapest method, broadband ultrasound attenuation, appears to perform as well as more expensive techniques such as dual energy x-ray absorptiometry (DXA).[37] Although DXA may be more appropriate for monitoring treatment in specialist centres, this monitoring function may be achieved at similar or lower cost using measurements of biochemical markers.[38] For use as a simple risk stratifying device, quantitative ultrasound (QUS) is likely to be more cost-effective than DXA due to its much reduced purchase price of £15 000 versus £60 000 in 1996. With respect to biochemical markers (such as urinary deoxypyridinoline) their price differential is not as great as that between QUS and DXA (£25 versus £40). However, the measurement of biochemical markers can be initiated sooner after the start of treatment (6 months compared with 24 months) and therefore, there is a greater possibility of reducing costs by avoiding giving therapeutic regimes to nonresponsive patients. However, we acknowledge that there is no formal cost analysis available of biochemical markers compared with DXA for monitoring response to therapy.

6. Conclusions and Future Economic Research

The 'bone field' is a relatively fast moving area at the present time with a number of new therapeutic treatments recently licensed or in the latter stages of phase III clinical trials. Furthermore, new methods of assessing risk, such as markers of bone turnover and improvements in current technologies to assess bone mass, may lead to a change in the relative cost effectiveness of treatment patterns. It is important, therefore, when new modes of treatment and assessment are evaluated clinically that a concurrent economic evaluation is undertaken.

In conclusion, osteoporosis constitutes a major public health problem, whether measured by the prevalence of reduced bone density in the general population, or by the incidence of age-related fractures. These fractures result from a complex interaction between bone strength and falling, and preventive strategies are available which can be directed at the entire population or at high risk individuals. The task of much current research is to validate the use of these preventive strategies and to better define the setting in which various approaches are most effective.

References

1. Anonymous. Consensus development conference diagnosis prophylaxis and treatment of osteoporosis. Am J Med 1993; 94: 646-50
2. Nevitt MC, Cummings SR. The Study of Osteoporotic Fractures Research Group. Type of fall and risk of hip and wrist fractures; the study of osteoporotic fractures. J Am Geriatr Soc 1993; 41: 1226-30
3. Cooper C, Melton LJ. Magnitude and impact of osteoporosis and fractures. In: Marcus R, Feldman D, Kelsey J, editors. Osteoporosis. San Diego: Academic Press Inc, 1996: 419-34
4. Cooper C, Melton LJ. Epidemiology of osteoporosis. Trends Endocrinol Metab 1992; 3: 224-29
5. Jacobsen SJ, Goldberg J, Miles TP, et al. Seasonal variation in the incidence of hip fracture among white persons aged 65 and older in the US, 1984-87. Am J Epidemiol 1991; 133: 996-1004
6. Maggi S, Kelsey JC, Litvak J, et al. Incidence of hip fractures in the elderly; a cross-national analysis. Osteoporosis Int 1991; 1: 232-41
7. Adebajo A, Cooper C, Evans JG. Fracture of the hip and distal forearm in West Africa and the United Kingdom. Age Ageing 1991; 20: 435-38
8. Jacobsen SJ, Goldberg J, Miles TP. Regional variation in the incidence of hip fracture in US white women aged 65 years and older. JAMA 1990; 264: 500-2
9. Cooper C, Campion G, Melton III LJ. Hip fractures in the elderly: a world-wide projection. Osteoporosis Int 1993; 2: 285-9
10. Cooper C, Atkinson EJ, O'Fallon WM, et al. The incidence of clinically diagnosed vertebral fracture: a population-based study in Rochester, Minnesota. J Bone Miner Res 1992; 7: 221-7
11. Riggs BL, Melton LJ. Evidence for two distinct syndromes of involutional osteoporosis. Am J Med 1993; 75: 899-901
12. Compston JE, Cooper C, Kanis JA. Bone densitometry in clinical practice. BMJ 1995; 310: 1507-10
13. Dennison E, Cooper C. The epidemiology of osteoporosis. Br J Clin Pract 1996; 50: 33-6
14. Kanis JA, the WHO Study Group. Assessment of fracture risk and its application to screening for postmenopausal osteoporosis. Synopsis of a WHO Report. Osteoporosis Int 1994; 4: 368-81
15. Felson DT, Zhang Y, Hannan M, et al. The effect of postmenopausal oestrogen therapy on bone density in elderly women. N Engl J Med 1993; 329: 1141-6
16. Dawson-Hughes B, Dallal G, Krall E, et al. A controlled trial of the effect of calcium supplementation on bone density in postmenopausal women. N Engl J Med 1990; 323: 878-83
17. Reid IR, Ames R, Evans M, et al. Effect of calcium supplementation on bone loss in postmenopausal women. N Engl J Med 1993; 328: 460-4
18. Chapuy M, Arlot M, Duboeuf F, et al. Vitamin D_3 and calcium to prevent hip fracture in the elderly. N Engl J Med 1992; 327: 1537-42
19. Storm T, Thamsborg G, Steiniche T, et al. Effect of intermittent cyclical etidronate therapy on bone mass and fracture rate in women with postmenopausal osteoporosis. N Engl J Med 1990; 322: 1265-71
20. Watts NB, Harris ST, Genant HK. Intermittent cyclical etidronate treatment of postmenopausal osteoporosis. N Engl J Med 1990; 323: 73-9
21. Adami S, Broggini M, Caruso I, et al. Treatment of postmenopausal osteoporosis with continuous daily oral alendronate in comparison to either placebo or intranasal salmon calcitonin. Osteoporosis Int 1993; Suppl. 3: S21-8
22. Riggs BL, Hodgson SF, O'Fallon WM, et al. Effect of fluoride treatment on the fracture rate in postmenopausal women with osteoporosis. N Engl J Med 1990; 322: 802-9
23. Kleerekoper M, Peterson EL, Nelson DA et al. A randomised trial of sodium fluoride as a treatment for postmenopausal osteoporosis. Osteoporosis Int 1991; 1: 155-61
24. Barlow DH. Advisory Group on Osteoporosis. London: Department of Health, 1994
25. Hollingworth W, Todd CJ, Parker MJ. The cost of treating hip fractures in the twenty-first century. J Public Health Med 1995; 17: 269-79
26. Torgerson DJ. The costs of treating osteoporotic fractures in the United Kingdom female population. IFSSD-WHO-EFFO Social and Economic Aspects of Osteoporosis Symposium; 1997 Dec 4-6; Liege, Belgium
27. Byford S, Torgerson DJ, Rafftery J. Cost of illness studies. BMJ. In press
28. Torgerson DJ, Reid DM. The economics of osteoporosis and its prevention. Pharmacoeconomics 1997; 11 (2): 126-38
29. Torgerson DJ, Gosden T, Reid DM. The economics of osteoporosis prevention. Trends Endocrinol Metab 1997; 8: 236-9

30. Cauley JA, Seeley DG, Ensrud K, et al. Estrogen replacement therapy and fractures in older women. Ann Intern Med 1995; 122: 9-16
31. Tosteson ANA, Rosenthal DI, Melton J, et al. Cost-effectiveness of screening perimenopausal white women for osteoporosis: bone densitometry and hormone replacement therapy. Ann Intern Med 1990; 113: 549-603
32. Francis RM, Anderson FH, Torgerson DJ. A comparison of the effectiveness and cost of treatment for vertebral fractures in women. Br J Rheumatol 1995; 34: 1167-71
33. Lauritzen JB, Petersen MM, Lund B. Effect of external hip protectors on hip fractures. Lancet 1993; 341: 11-3
34. Ekman A, Mallmin H, Michanelsson K, et al. External hip protectors to prevent osteoporotic fractures. Lancet 1997; 350: 563-4
35. Schroder HM, Petersen KK, Erlansen M. Occurrence and incidence of second hip fracture. Clin Orthop 1993; 289: 166-9
36. Lauritzen JB, Hindso K, Singh G. Cost effectiveness of external hip protectors [abstract]. Calcif Tissue Int 1997; 61 (6): 501
37. Bauer DC, Gluer CC, Cauley JA, et al. Broadband ultrasound attenuation predicts fracture strongly and independently of densitometry in older women. Arch Intern Med 1997; 157: 629-34
38. Eastell R, Blumsohn A. Biochemical markers of bone turnover in osteoporosis. In: Compston JE, editor. Osteoporosis. London: Royal College of Physicians of London, 1996: 55-64

Correspondence: Prof. *C. Cooper,* MRC Environmental Epidemiology Unit, Southampton General Hospital, Southampton, SO16 6YD, England.